CHRISTMAS IN HOLLYWOOD: TOXIC RIDDLE FOR THE TOXIC DETECTIVE

An Indian Society of Toxicology Initiative

Dr Vivekanshu Verma
Dr Vijay Vasudev Pillay
Dr Shiv Rattan Kochar
Dr Prateek Rastogi

Poison Control Centre
Amrita Institute of Medical Science,
Ponekkara, P. O, Kochi, Kerala - 682041.

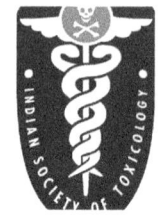

Copyright © 2020 © Indian Society of Toxicology

All rights reserved

The characters and events portrayed in this book are fictitious.

Any similarity to real persons, living or dead, is coincidental and not intended by the author.

No part of this book may be reproduced, or stored in a retrieval system, or transmitted in any form or by any means, electronic, mechanical, photocopying, recording, or otherwise, without express written permission of the publisher.

ISBN: 9798586294586

Cover design by: Vishwendra Verma
Library of Congress Control Number: 2018675309
Printed in the Poison Control Centre
Amrita Institute of Medical Science,
Ponekkara, P. O, Kochi, Kerala - 682041.

We dedicate this book on Toxic Riddles to all the Toxicology Nurses, Medical students, Senior residents, and fellows from the school of medicine, nursing, law, police academy and pharmacy, who strongly feel that Riddle solving approach is a must for all involved healthcare providers who strive to be the best caretakers of their patients suffering from poisoning, drug overdose or intoxication.

We hope that this book will aid all young budding toxicologists' quest to excellence, who want to practice their professional skills conscientiously and fearlessly and are keen to promote quality in healthcare of poisoning victims.

We are also grateful to our teachers, parents, elders and seniors for their blessings, constant motivation and support, in materializing the dream cum true of compiling a textbook on toxicology.

We wish to dedicate this treatise to Late Dr Chiranji Lal Verma, who was an expert surgeon & guided in motivating us to become, what we,are today.

In last, We would also dedicate this book to cute little niece Heeral, a bundle of joy, without whom, this would not have been possible.

CONTENTS

Title Page
Copyright
Dedication
Preface
201st Toxic Riddles in Rhyme   6
ARE CHRISTMAS TREES POISONOUS?   8
RIDDLE ANALYSIS   10
Description: 14
Clinical Findings: 15
Family: Aquifoliaceae   16
Common Names: 17
SO AM I, LACKS OPAQUE A, UNSAFE TO HANDLE,   19
NOW ITS FROSTY WIND WINTERS, DON'T FEEL ALONE,   21
LET CHILDREN GATHER TO CELEBRATE, DANCE & DINE   24
HOLIDAY   26
HOLLY-BOY & AN IVY-GIRL   27
CHIMNEY-SWEEPS BY HOLLY's BRANCH   30
BIRDLIME BY HOLLIES   32
HEALING WITH HOLLIES   34
EARTH STOOD HARD AS IRON, WATER FREEZE AS STONE   36
STAR AND ANGELS DELIVER BY THE HOLY SACRED SIGN   37

SING CHRISTMAS CAROL FOR LORD JESUS'S BIRTHDAY	40
SANTA CLAUS TO INCARNATE FILLS WISHES DIVINE,	41
WITH HOLLY TREES GROW GREEN & SOW, TO LAY,	43
Decorating for Christmas with Holly	44
ORIENTAL HOLLY	45
GIFT HIDDEN IN SOCKS, U DECORATE TREE MINE,	47
WE DECK UP UR HOUSES AS FRESH AS YOU SAY	49
MERRILY GATHER MASS CROWD ROUND MY TREE	50
HOLLY WOOD CABINET WORK, TO WHIP-HANDLE	52
I OFTEN DISPLAY "A" PYRAMIDAL SPIKE SPREE	53
AS THE WHOLLY BRIGHT GIFTS HANG TO DANGLE	56
ILEX FLOWERS	59
FRUITS OF HOLLY	61
PEEPS THROUGH TREES WITH BERRIES OF RED,	64
LEGEND OF RED BERRIES	66
PYRENES OF HOLLY	67
CHEMICAL PROPERTIES	68
LEAVES OF BURNISHED GREEN SPIKED ANGLE,	72
HOLLY'S HERBAL TEA	76
HOLLYWOOD- WHAT'S IN NAME	79
HOLLY WOOD's CUP DRINKS CURED TOTALLY	82
JOLLY's TOOTHACHE CURED BY HOLLY	83
BARK to disinfect	84
HOLLIES	85
MY ATTRACTIVE FRUITS ARE HARMFUL, AS I SAID	86
Toxins	87
FATAL DOSE	88
FATAL PERIOD	89

HOLLY'S MELANCHOLY	90
Holiday plants with toxic misconceptions	91
Diagnosis	92
First-aid measures and management principles	93
AND SO NEVER GET LURED TO MY BEAUTIFUL HUE,	95
WARN UNTO MY TOXIC RED BERRIES, LIKE YEW	97
FOR KIDS & PETS MIGHT ATE TO MANHANDLE,	98
Twin Hollies	99
Ipecac in Holly	100
AS BERRIES ARE FATAL, TURNS CYANOTIC BLUE	101
IT'S NATURE'S GIFT, TO PROTECT AGAINST VANDAL	102
BEVERAGE	105
AS BERRIES CAUSES CARDIAC ARREST, IF ADDED TO BREW	109
TEN-IN= Tannin	111
CONICAL ARROW HEAD WERE POISONED AMPLE	112
MY TOXIN ACTS LIKE DIGITALIS IN ECG TO SKEW	113
BETTER BUY MY ARTIFICIAL TREES GLOW CANDLE	115
AND ENJOY SAFE FESTIVALS, HAPPY YEAR, NEW	117
How can you tell an American holly from English Holly?	124
THE CHRISTMAS HOLLY Poem by ELIZA COOK (1818-1889)	125
Charles Dickens -A Christmas Carol	129
	131
Bibliography & Suggested Reading:	
	133
Our Books on Toxicology	
Contributors:	137

PREFACE

Toxicology riddle solving is neither art nor science, but rather a craft.

It requires a commitment to excellence from a craftsman.

Paying it forward is part of the deal.

This work is our attempt to share what we've learned about Medical Toxicology with the next generation.

Writing a book is not an easy task, and neither is being a Toxicologist.

    Toxic Riddles narrated in Rhymes;
    During Terror of Corona times;
    By Toxic Detective for solving Crimes;
    On Indian Society of Toxicology (IST)'s Paradigms;
    Happy Learning!

DR VIVEKANSHU VERMA FIST

Christmas in Hollywood: Toxic Riddle for the Toxic Detective

An Indian Society of Toxicology Initiative

For Toxic Detectives, Crime Scene Investigators (CSi), Toxicologists, Police Officers, CID & CBI officers, Lawyers, Judges, Magistrates, Legal counsels, Law Students, Forensic Scientists, Doctors, Toxicology Nurses & Emergency Paramedics

Dr Vivekanshu Verma, MBBS, Postgraduate Diploma in Forensic Medicine & Toxicology, Fellow of Indian Society of Toxicology, Associate consultant, Emergency & Trauma care, Medanta-The Medicity, Gurugram. Honorary Toxicology Expert, Central Bureau of Investigation

Dr Vijay Vasudev Pillay, MBBS, MD Forensic Medicine & Toxicology, Chief, Poison Control Centre, Professor & Head, Forensic Medicine & Toxicology, Amrita School of Medicine, Amrita Vishwa Vidyapeetham, Cochin, Kerala

Dr Shiv Rattan Kochar, MBBS, MD Forensic Medicine & Toxicology, Senior Professor, Forensic Medicine. Chief Vigilance Officer, Metro MANAS Arogya Sadan Heart Care & Multispecialty Hospital, Directorate of Medical Education, Jaipur (Rajasthan)

Dr Prateek Rastogi, MBBS,MD, PGDMLE, PGDCFS, PGCMNCPA, PGCTM, Dip. Cyber Law, FAGE, FAIMER Fellow (MUFILIPE-Manipal), Former President, Indian Society of Toxicology(2018-19), Professor, Department of Forensic Medicine & Toxicology, Kasturba Medical College, Mangalore, Karnataka

ISBN: 9798586294586

©2020 Indian Society of Toxicology

2U 🎄 Toxic 🌿 Riddles 🎋 in 🎅 Rhymes 🎶
Now 👻 its Frosty wind 🌬 winters, 😨 don't feel 😔 alone,
Let Children 👨‍👩‍👧 gather to 🎉 celebrate, 💃 dance & 🍖 dine
Earth 🌍 stood hard as iron, 💧 Water ❄ freeze as stone
Star ⭐ & Angels 👼 🕊 deliver by the holy 🙏 sacred sign
Sing 🎤 Christmas carol   for 👑 Lord Jesus's birthday
Santa Claus 🎅 to incarnate 🌼 fills 🎁 wishes ✨ Divine,
With Holly ⚡ trees 🌲 grow 🌱 green & sow, to lay, 🎄
Gift 🎁 hidden in 🧦 socks, U 🎀 decorate 🌲 tree mine,
We 🙌 deck up 🏠 Ur houses 🌟 as fresh 🍃 as you say
Merrily 👪 gather mass 👥 crowd round my 🎄 tree
🎬 Holly-wood 🪵 cabinet work, to 🏒 whip-handle
I often 🔴 display "A" pyramidal 🎄 spike 🎉 spree
As the 🕯 wholly bright gifts 🎁 hang to dangle
Peeps 👀 through 🌲 trees with berries 🍒 of red,
Leaves 🍃 of burnished 🍀 green spiked 🍃 angle,
My attractive 🍓 fruits are ⚠ harmful, as I said
And so 😈 never get lured to my beautiful 🎨 hue,
So am I, lacks 💀 opaque A, unsafe 🤚 to handle,
Warn ⚠ unto my toxic 🍒 red berries, like 💀 yew
For kids & 🐕 pets might ate to 🐾 manhandle,
As berries 🍒 are fatal, turns cyanotic 😨 blue
It's nature's 🎁 gift, to protect against 🦹 vandal
As causes 💔 cardiac arrest, if added to 🍵 brew
Conical arrow head ⭕ were poisoned 🎯 ample
My toxin 👽 acts like 💊 digitalis in ECG to 📉 skew
Better 🛒 buy 🎄 artificial 🎄 trees, glow as 🕯 candle
And 🎊 enjoy 🎉 safe festivals, happy year, ✨ New

Toxic Hint to Riddle No. 201:

What is the toxicological significance of Christmas Tree & related mythological connection to Hollywood ?

201ST TOXIC RIDDLES IN RHYME

Now its Frosty wind winters, don't feel alone,
Let Children gather to celebrate, dance & dine
Earth stood hard as iron, Water freeze as stone
Star and Angels deliver by the holy sacred sign
Sing Christmas carol for Lord Jesus's birthday
Santa Claus to incarnate fills wishes Divine,
With Holly trees grow green & sow, to lay,
Gift hidden in socks, U decorate tree mine,
We deck up Ur houses as fresh as you say
Merrily gather mass crowd round my tree
Holly wood cabinet work, to whip-handle
I often display "A" pyramidal spike spree
As the wholly bright gifts hang to dangle
Peeps through trees with berries of red,
Leaves of burnished green spiked angle,
My attractive fruits are harmful, as I said
And so never get lured to my beautiful hue,
So am I, lacks opaque A, unsafe to handle,
Warn unto my toxic red berries, like yew

For kids & pets might ate to manhandle,
As berries are fatal, turns cyanotic blue
It's nature's gift, to protect against vandal
As causes cardiac arrest, if added to brew
Conical arrow head were poisoned ample
My toxin acts like digitalis in ECG to skew
Better buy my artificial trees with candle
And enjoy safe festivals, happy year, New

ARE CHRISTMAS TREES POISONOUS?

Christmas trees such as firs, pines, and cedar are mildly poisonous, sometimes causing drooling in pets and vomiting in children.

The good news is that a child or pet would have to eat quite a bit to become sick and people and pets usually don't like to eat Christmas trees.

The toxicity of the tree may be increased if it has been sprayed with a fire retardant.

Although the oil from Christmas trees can irritate the mouth and skin, the real concern is that if a small child or pet eats only a few needles, which are almost impossible to digest, the needles could puncture or obstruct part of their intestinal tract.

Eating parts of an artificial tree is also dangerous since there can be toxins in the tree material and pieces of the tree can cause intestinal obstructions.

Another thing we tend to forget is the water the tree is sitting in to keep it looking fresh.

This water may contain preservatives, pesticides, fertilizers, or some people even put aspirin into it.

Cover the water dish so that cats and dogs don't drink from it and small children don't play in it.

RIDDLE ANALYSIS

The word holly is often used in the name of plants that do not belong to the genus Ilex.

These plants may have holly-like foliage or resemble holly in some other way, or they may simply make use of the word holly to create an interesting common name such as hollyhock.

Holly is a small tree or shrub that will grow up to 15 m tall and carries scarlet red berries approximately 10 mm in diameter.

These shrubs are most commonly used as holiday decorations, although they can be found in gardens.

Holly exposure accounts for the 3rd highest rate of genus-specific human plant exposure calls in 2010, with 877.

Botanically Holly is classified as Ilex species.

Common Name	Scientific Name
African holly	*Solanum giganteum*
Arizona holly	*Photinia serratifolia*
box holly	*Ruscus aculeatus*
Braun's holly fern	*Polystichum braunii*
California holly	*Heteromeles arbutifolia, Photinia arbutifolia,*
California holly grape	*Mahonia lomariifolia*
Chinese holly	*Osmanthus heterophyllus*
Chinese holly grape	*Mahonia japonica*
Cuban holly	*Atriplex hymenelytra*
desert holly	*Atriplex hymenelytra*
dwarf holly	*Malpighia coccigera*
false holly	*Osmanthus heterophyllus*
holly berry vine	*Lycium chinensis*
holly cherry	*Prunus ilicifolia*
holly fern	*Polystichum falcatum, P. lonchitis*
holly grape	*Mahonia aquifolium*
holly oak	*Quercus chrysolepis, Q. ilex*
holly scale	*Atriplex hymenelytra*
holly xylosma	*Xylosma heterophylla*
hollyhock, sea	*Eryngium maritimum, Hibiscus palustris*
holly-leaved ashberry	*Mahonia bealei*
holly-leaved barberry	*Berberis ilicifolia*
holly-leaved cherry	*Prunus laurocerasus*
holly-leaved olive	*Osmanthus aquifolium*
holly-leaved osmanthus	*Osmanthus heterophyllus*
Japanese holly	*Mahonia japonica*
miniature holly	*Malpighia coccigera*

Common Name	Scientific Name
Chinese spiny holly	*I. cornuta*
Christmas holly	*I. aquifolium, I. opaca*
christdorn	*I. aquifolium*
citronnien	*I. nitida*
citronnier	*I. sideroxyloides*
citronnier-montagne	*I. dioica*
cogolin	*I. sideroxyloides*
common holly	*I. aquifolium*
congonha	*I. affinis, I. conocarpa, I. cuyabensis, I. paltorioides, paraguariensis, I. vitis-idaea*
congonha do campo	*I. affinis*
congonhas minda	*I. dumosa*
congonhinha	*I. chamaedryfolia, I. congonhinha*
congoroba	*I. amara*
cueri de sapo	*I. urbaniana*
cuero de sapo	*I. nitida*
Curtiss's holly	*I. curtissii*
Cuthbert's holly	*I. cuthbertii*
dahoon holly	*I. cassine*
deciduous holly	*I. decidua*
deciduous yaupon holly	*I. decidua*
deer-berry	*I. vomitoria*
diusa	*I. dipyrena*
dogberry	*I. verticillata*
droopbead holly	*I. geniculata*
dune holly	*I. cumulicola*
Dutch holly	a group within *I.* × *altaclerensis*
Dutch-English holly	a group within *I.* × *altaclerensis*
dwarf box holly	*I. crenata*
eastern holly	*I. opaca*
Egham holly	*I. aquifolium* 'Heterophylla Aureomarginata'

emetic holly	*I. vomitoria*
English holly	*I. aquifolium*
European holly	*I. aquifolium*
evergreen cassena	*I. vomitoria*
evergreen cassine	*I. vomitoria*
false alder	*I. verticillata*
fan cha shu	*I. corallina*
farmer variegated holly	*I. aquifolium* 'Variegated'
feverbush	*I. verticillata*
fuiri-inu-tsugi	*I. crenata* f. *luteo-variegata*
fuiri-soyogo	*I. pedunculosa* f. *variegata*
furin Holly	*I. geniculata*
furin-ume-modoki	*I. geniculata*
furi machi no ki	*I.* 'Green Shadow'
gading	*I. macrophylla*
gallberry	*I. glabra*

DESCRIPTION:

Ilex species are evergreen trees with alternate, stiff leathery leaves.

Flowers are small and white.

Fruits are usually bright red at maturity.

Toxic Part: The fruit is poisonous.

Toxin: Saponins.

CLINICAL FINDINGS:

Most ingestions result in little or no toxicity. The saponins are poorly absorbed, but with large exposures gastrointestinal symptoms of nausea, vomiting, abdominal cramping, and diarrhea may occur.

Allergic sensitization to this plant is common and can cause severe allergic reactions.

The leaves are nontoxic, and those of some species (e.g., Ilex paraguariensis, or Maté) are brewed as a beverage for their content of caffeine (or other xanthines).

FAMILY: AQUIFOLIACEAE

Ilex aquifolium L.

Ilex opaca Aiton

Ilex vomitoria Aiton

COMMON NAMES:

Ilex aquifolium: Holly, English Holly, European Holly, Oregon Holly

Ilex opaca: American Holly, Waysides Christmas tree

Ilex vomitoria: Yaupon, Appalachian or Carolina Tea, Cassena, Deer Berry,

Emetic Holly, Evergreen Cassena, Indian Black Drink.

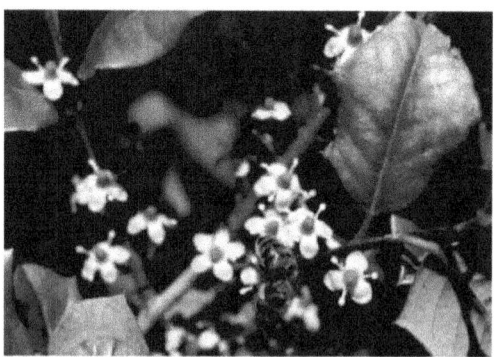

Ilex opaca, flowering branch (above)

Ilex opaca, branches with fruit (below)

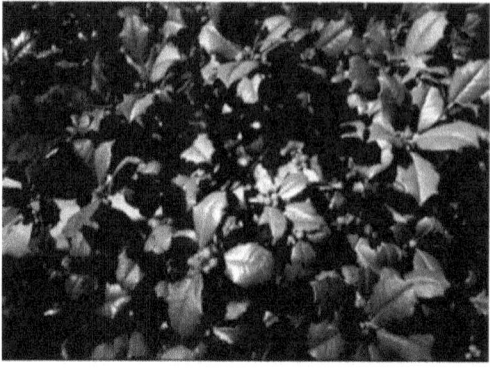

Figure 1. Ilex opaca. Image source: Individual Plants. In: Handbook of Poisonous and Injurious Plants. (2007) Springer, Boston, MA.

SO AM I, LACKS OPAQUE A, UNSAFE TO HANDLE,

decoding

I, lacks opaque = Ilex opaca (homophonic)

Ilex opaca or American holly is an evergreen tree growing throughout the Atlantic section of the United States.

Holly days = Holidays (homophonic)

There are few groups of trees and shrubs that possess such a fascinating and diverse background as do the plants belonging to the genus Ilex or, as they are more commonly called, hollies.

There are 2 commonly distributed forms of the holly in the United States (U.S.): the English holly (Ilex aquifolium) and the American Holly (Ilex opaca).

English and American holly are not to be confused with the South American Ilex species, Ilex paraguariensi and Ilex guayusa, which are commonly used to make teas and other drinks for their reported antioxidant properties and caffeine content.

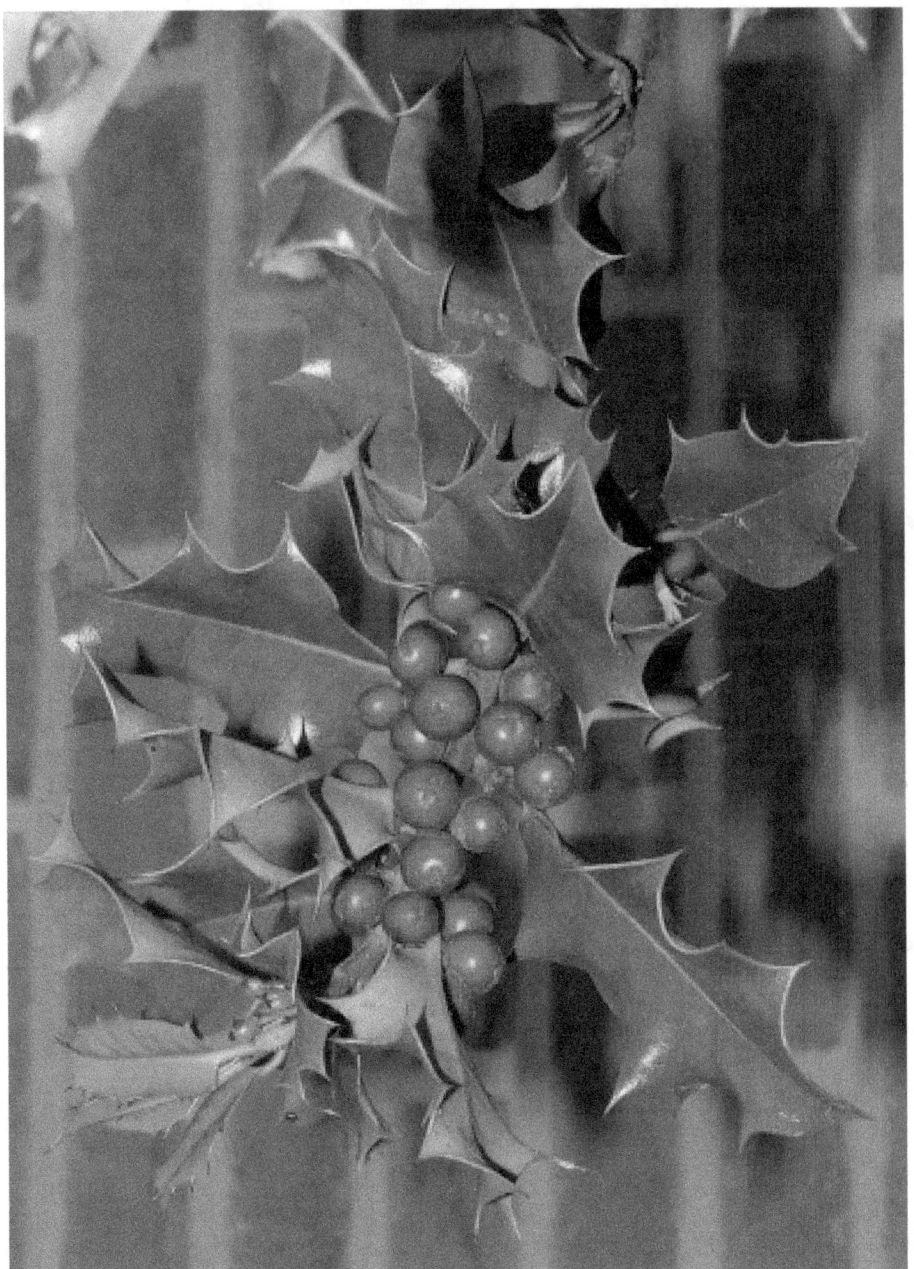

Figure 2. Holly (Ilex aquifolium and opaca) Evens ZN, Stellpflug SJ. Holiday plants with toxic misconceptions. West J Emerg Med. 2012 Dec;13(6):538-42.

NOW ITS FROSTY WIND WINTERS, DON'T FEEL ALONE,

Home Alone movie themed around the Christmas vacations, in which all family members leave for outing, and the child in left alone at home, who protects himself & his home from thieves, and in last decorates Christmas Tree, to find his wishes fulfilled.

Home Alone (1990) movie was made in Hollywood, USA.

Thus Holly-wood is related to Holly tree, found in USA, to celebrate Christmas, by decorating it.

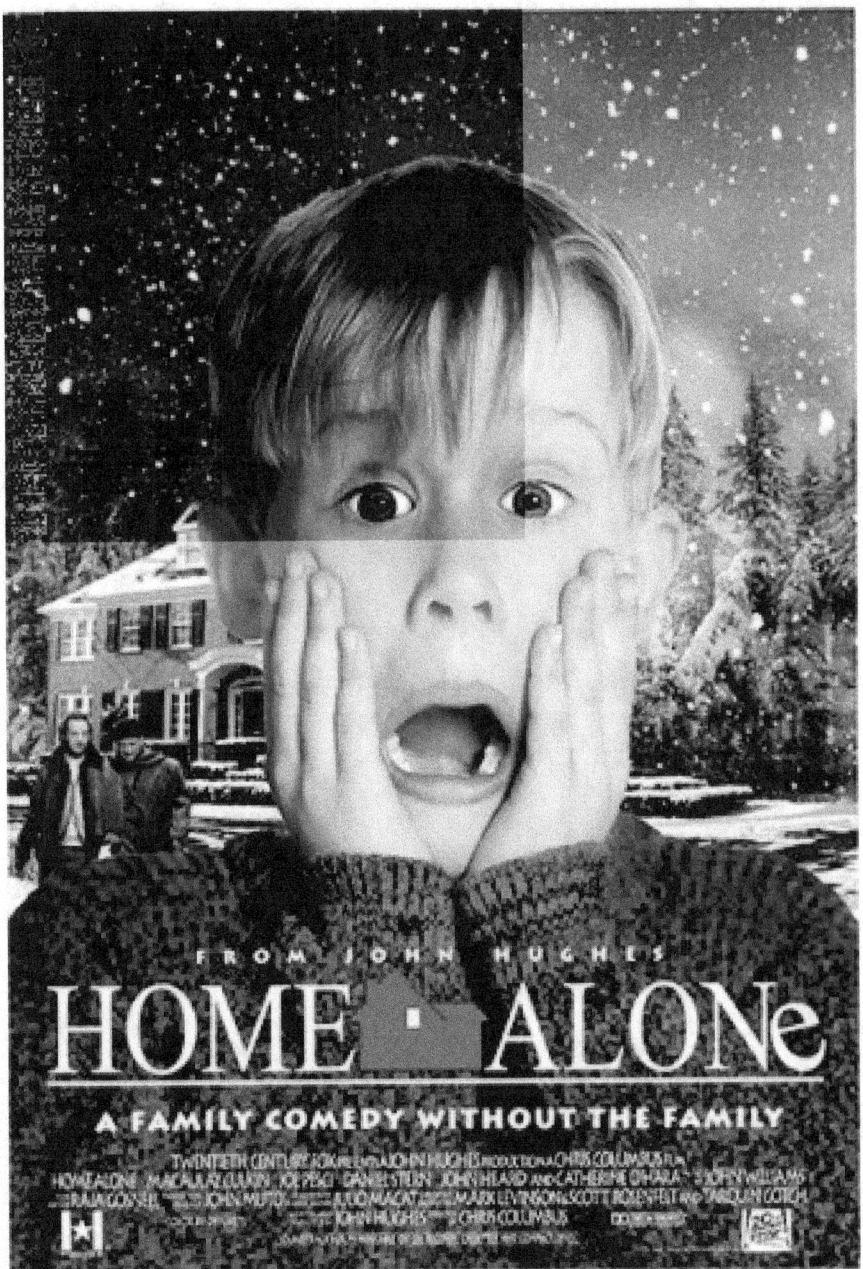

Figure 3. Home Alone (1990) movie made in Hollywood, USA

In the old floral vocabularies, mistletoe represented the ability to overcome difficulties, while holly stood for foresight; a bouquet of the two plants carried this message:

"By foresight you will surmount your difficulties."

LET CHILDREN GATHER TO CELEBRATE, DANCE & DINE

Of all such festivals, none is perhaps more widely known than that of the Saturnalia, which took place in December, the last month of the Roman year, about the time of our present Christmas.

The Saturnalia commemorated the good King Saturn, god of sowing and husbandry, during whose reign no war was rife, the fields and flocks produced abundantly, no individuals were bound in slavery, and the world was a most pleasurable place in which to live.

During the great feast of Saturnalia, the Romans sent holly boughs along with a gift to their friends as token of their good wishes and as emblems of the esteem in which they held them.

It is from this custom that historians consider holly to be symbolic of goodwill and for this reason that we decorate our homes and churches with this colorful greenery during the holidays.

About a Nurse

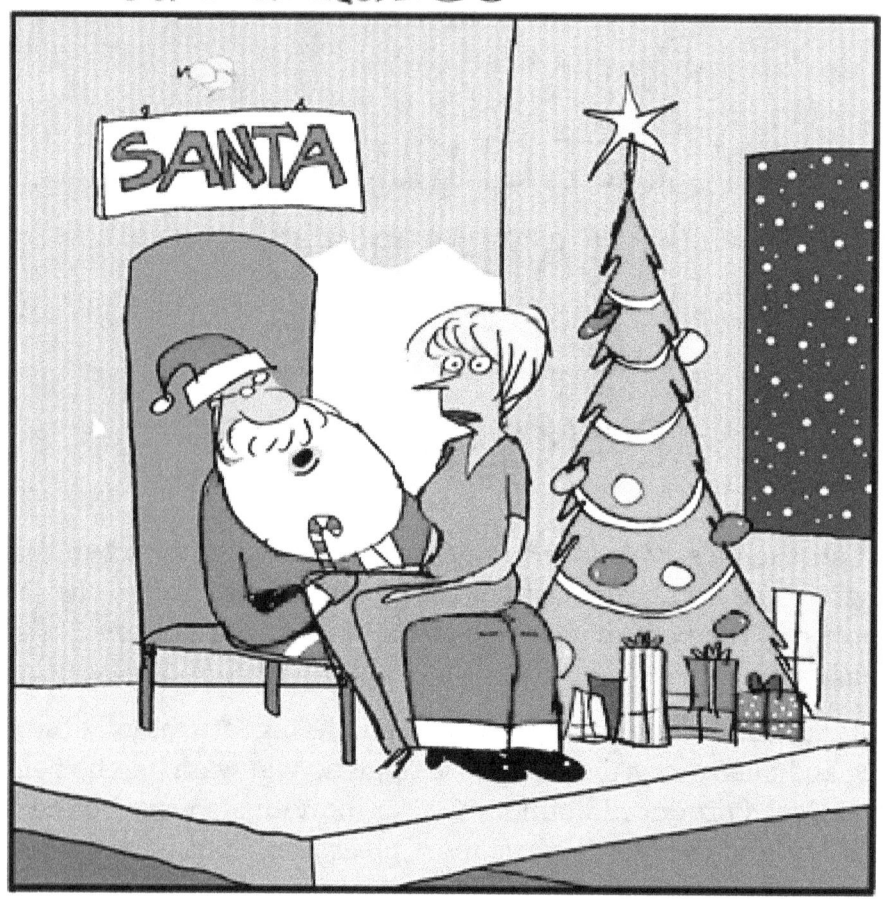

"I'm sorry, but I can't give you holidays off, or a social life. Would you settle for a candy cane?"

HOLIDAY

Holly = Holy = Holi (sound alike - Homophonic)

The word Holiday, might have originated from the Holly plant, decorated in Christmas, bringing Holidays.

Emergency Health care providers like paramedics, nurses, doctors & toxicologists are posted on special duties on rotation, during holidays.

Thus they filled burnt out & stressed, as they can't chill out with friends & family unlike others in public.

HOLLY-BOY & AN IVY-GIRL

In old traditional English Shrovetide dances, the last merry-making period before the observance of Lent there often appeared a holly-boy and an ivy-girl.

The holly was supposed to be male and to personify the steadfast and the holy, while the ivy, because of its clinging and embracing nature, was symbolical of a maiden love and friendship.

In some areas of England it was traditional for the girls to make chains of holly to burn on Shrove Tuesday, the boys retaliating with ropes of ivy (Dallimore 1908).

JACK IN THE GREEN

The observance of May Day, with its poles and dances, has long been a traditional custom of the spring festivals of European peasants.

This is a remnant of the ancient worship of the benevolent tree spirits and of the necessity each spring of paying homage to them to ensure the fertility of the fields and flocks in the coming year.

> Often, the spirit was represented by a pole, a freshly cut tree, a branch, a flower, a vegetable, a person, or some combination of the above, like a bough-bedecked mummer.

Jack-in-the-Green, so Sir James Frazer wrote, is the best-known example of the latter.

Encased in a wicker work covered with holly and ivy and surmounted by a crown of flowers and ribbons, he dances on May Day at the head of a troop of fellow chimney-sweeps, all collecting gifts of pennies.

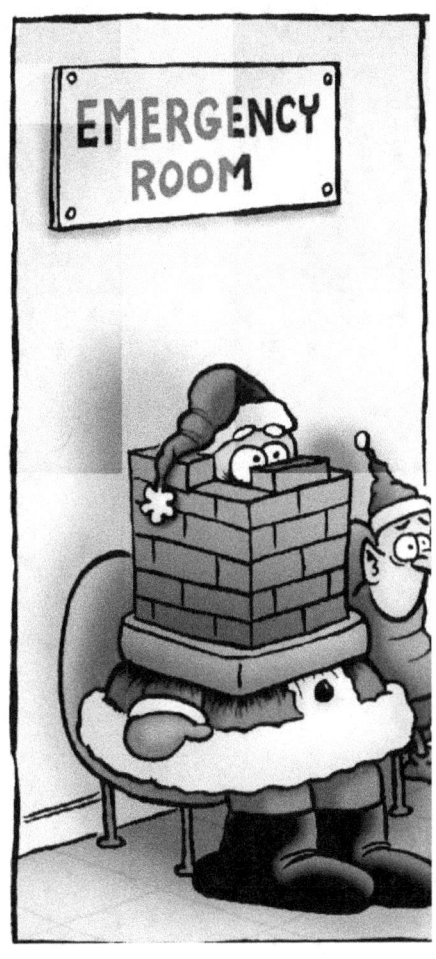

Figure 4. Its common myth that Santa Claus stucks in Chimney, if not kept cleaned, depicted in cartoon. Image source: Randy McIlwaine via CartoonStock.

CHIMNEY-SWEEPS BY HOLLY'S BRANCH

Here should be mentioned the preference of the chimney-sweeps, for branches of holly in cleaning the chimneys of London, and the tradition that all flues must be cleaned by New Year's Eve to permit an easy exit for all household evils.

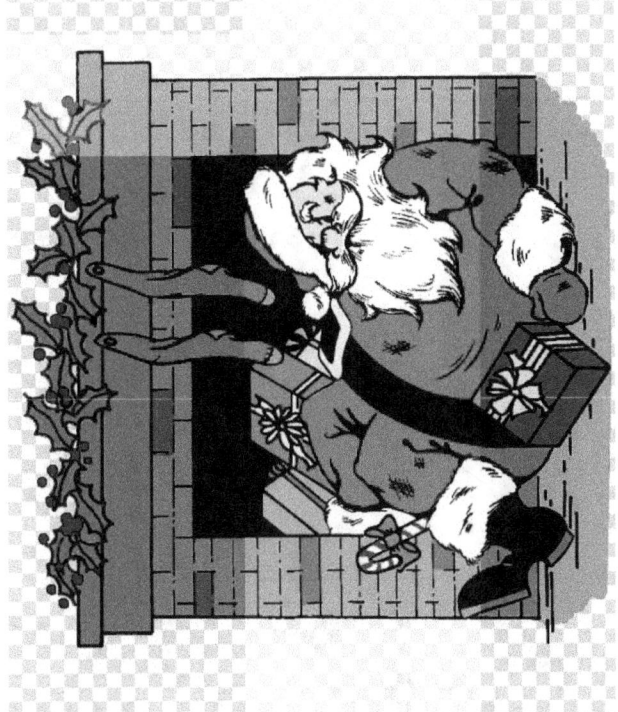

Figure 5. Hollies, Santa & Chimney as path filled with gifts, as per childhood stories in fairy tales & mythology

BIRDLIME BY HOLLIES

Of all the unusual customs concerning English hollies, perhaps none is more curious than the use of the bark in making birdlime.

This mucilaginous substance was spread on branches and other places where birds were accustomed to roost.

> In the days before firearms, there was no easier way of trapping the ingredients for a tasty sparrow pot pie.
>
> Birdlime was also used for keeping snails, insects, and other vermin from climbing fruit trees and invading gardens.
>
> In some provinces of China, bark of the beautiful *Ilex latifolia* is used for the same purposes.

> The bark of the holly was gathered in midsummer and boiled in spring water for twelve hours.
> On cooling, the inner green bark was separated from the rest and laid aside in a cool cellar for a fortnight, whence it became a perfect mucilage.
> It was then pounded fine in a mortar, washed in a stream of running water, boiled with a third part of capon or goose grease to prevent the birdlime from freezing in winter.

The folklore recorded here relates only to very few of the hundreds of hollies believed to occur in various parts of the world.

As these species gradually become introduced to the Americas, and as their folklore successively becomes known, a most exciting story is surely to be unfolded.

HEALING WITH HOLLIES

Among the many old and curious beliefs associated with healing was the idea that diseases could be transferred to trees and plants, especially by passing the patient through an arch or hoop of the branches, or through a cleft in the trunk of a tree. In almost every country of the world, this superstition could be found.

In England, ruptured children, or those with rickets, were passed through fissures of tree trunks, often of holly.

To ensure success, the tree could never before have been used for this purpose. The trunk was split from east to west; the youngster was passed through by a maiden and received by a boy on the other side.

Sometimes this was repeated three times; sometimes, too the child had to be thrust through head first for the charm to work; at other times, the feet had to be the foremost part of the body.

When the passing through ceremony was completed, the split that had been held open with wedges, was allowed to spring together, and the wound bound and plastered up with clay.

As the gash gradually healed, so did the youngster's rupture in a like manner.

> The largest-known American holly tree was similarly used to cure the rupture of a boy some forty years ago in North Carolina. The Russians used holly trees in a somewhat similar manner for curing tuberculosis.

EARTH STOOD HARD AS IRON, WATER FREEZE AS STONE

Much of our present-day folklore of medicines, superstitions, and Christmas customs comes from the practices and beliefs of the early Britons, which can be traced further to the Druids, an order of priests, teachers, philosophers, and astronomers of ancient Britain and Gaul, who lived some two thousand years ago.

The Druids believed that the sun never deserted the holly tree (Ilex aquifolium) and therefore that the holly was a sacred plant.

It was their custom to decorate the inside of their dwelling places with evergreens in which the woodland spirits would take refuge from the rigors of winter.

STAR AND ANGELS DELIVER BY THE HOLY SACRED SIGN

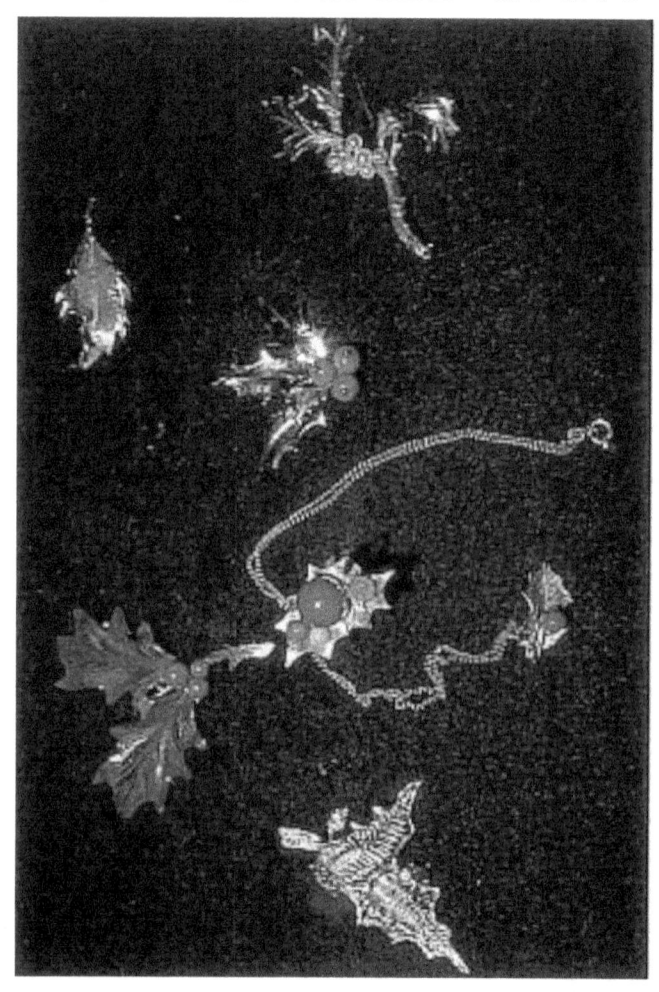

Figure 6. Holly jewelry. Photo by Barton Bauer Sr.

Holly has long been symbolic of Christmas.

The name is believed to be a corruption of the word *holy*, although many historians differ on the point. William Turner, the earliest English writer on plants, in his herbal of 1568 called the tree *Holy* and *Holytree*.

In parts of Italy, sprigs of holly were used to decorate mangers in commemoration of the infant savior.

In Germany, holly is called *Christdorn*, the thorn woven into the crown of crucifixion.

Legend has it that the berries of holly were once yellow, but, being stained from the wounds of Christ, have ever since remained red.

Among the old Pennsylvania Dutch, the holly berry represented the blood of Christ issuing from His wounds, and the white flowers of the holly tree were symbolic of the purity in which He was conceived.

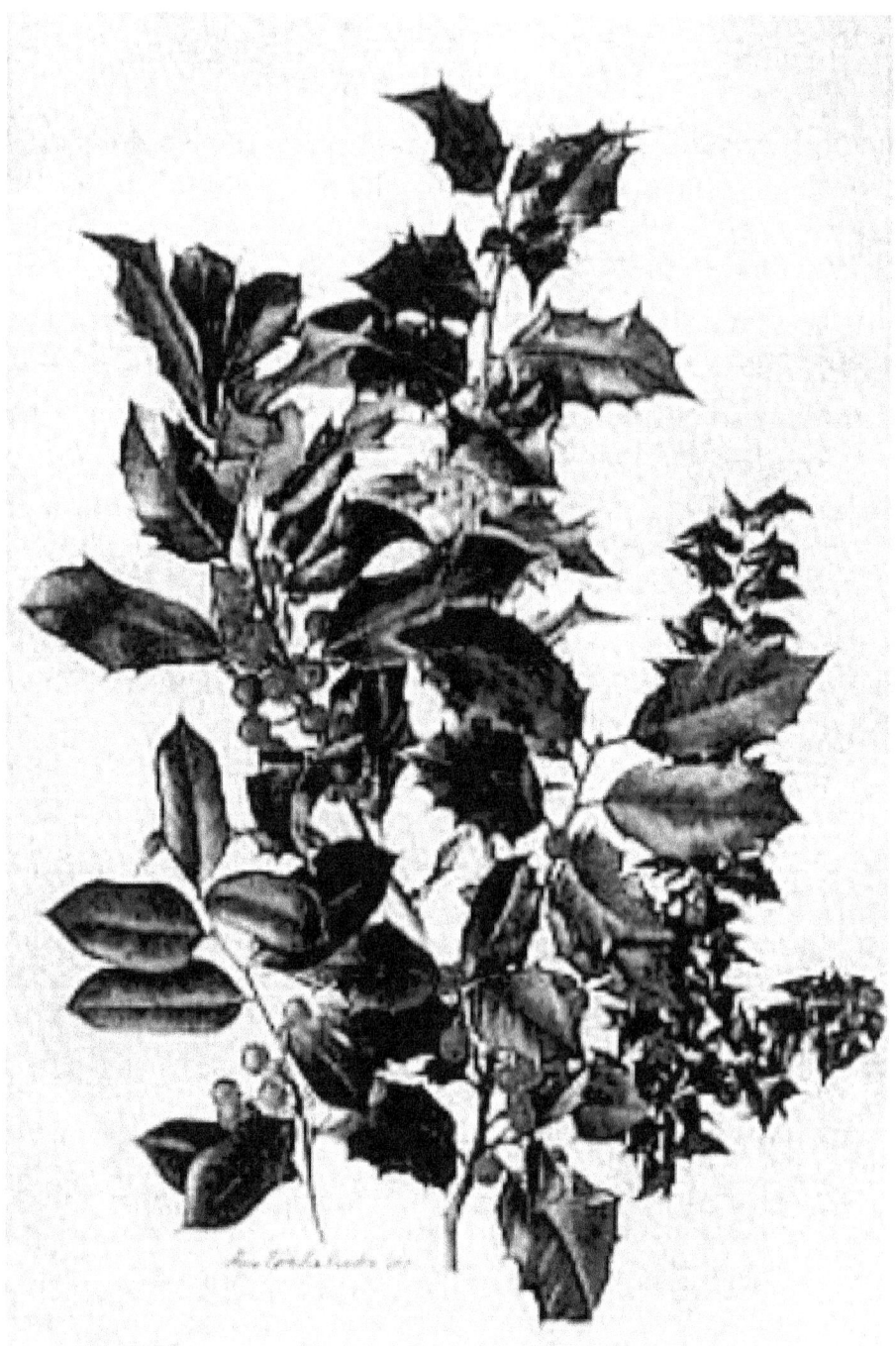

Figure 7. Christmas card with holly design. Photo by Fred Galle.

SING CHRISTMAS CAROL FOR LORD JESUS'S BIRTHDAY

Since the days of the Romans, the Greeks, the Druids, and the Indians of the Americas, holly has played an exciting part in medicine and magic, science and superstition, and legend and lore.

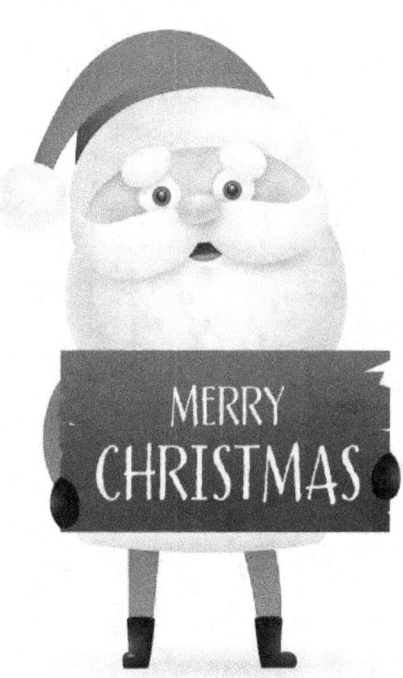

SANTA CLAUS TO INCARNATE FILLS WISHES DIVINE,

About a Nursing Student

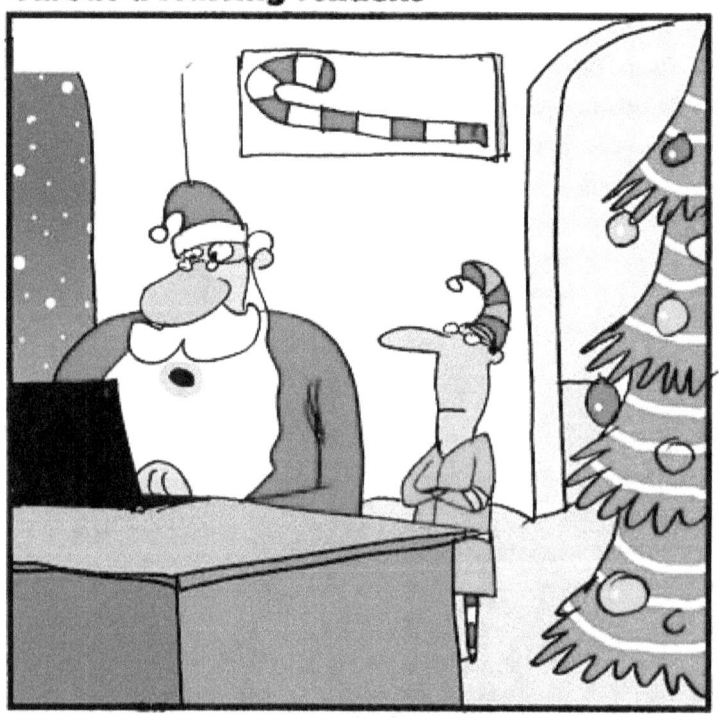

"*I can always tell who the nursing students are. All they ask for is sleep, time and money.*"

Figure 8. Most Nurses & doctors wish to have sleep, holidays & increment in salaries from Santa Claus on Xmas in Hospitals around artificial Christmas tree. Image source: www.allnurses.com

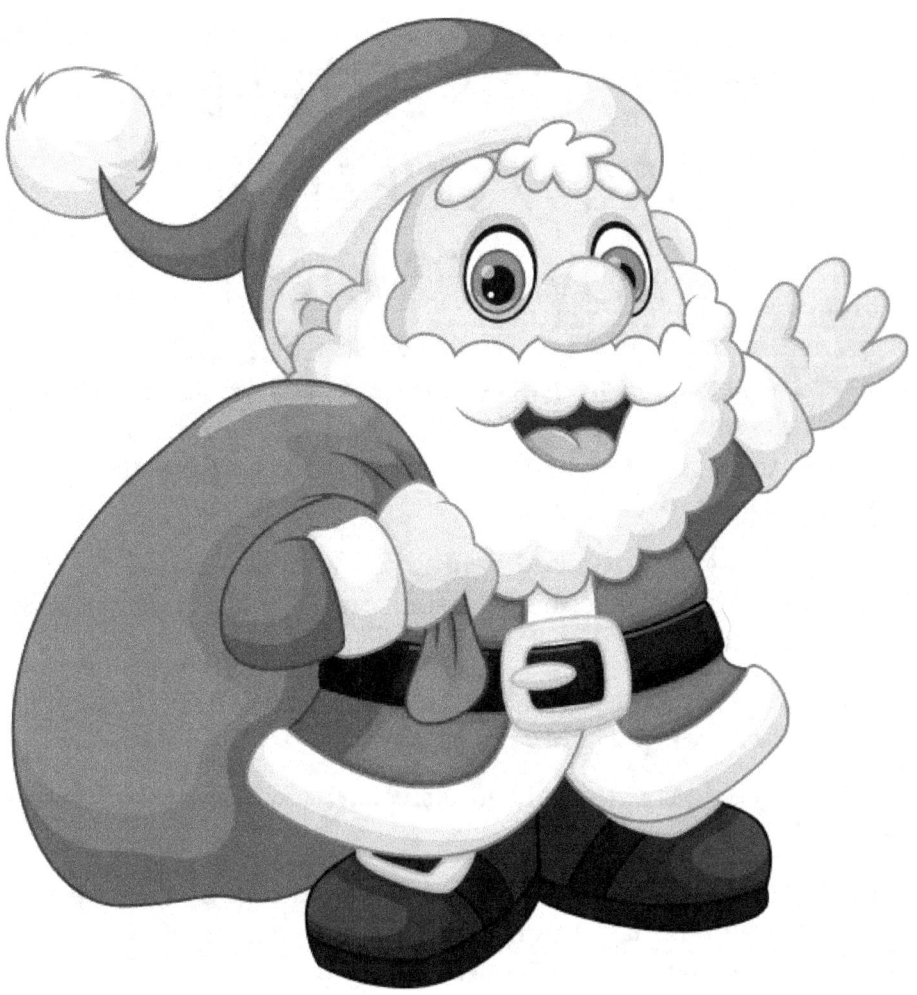

WITH HOLLY TREES GROW GREEN & SOW, TO LAY,

A branch of holly adorned with a cluster of bright red berries evokes thoughts of Christmas as readily as Santa and Rudolph. Ilex opaca (American holly) projects the image all of us carry as the epitome of holly; however, other hollies will create bolder and varied looks for decorations.

Just a sprig of holly tucked behind a brass candlestick, or tied with a red ribbon to a sconce, or stuck on a window pane will put the finishing touch of Christmas decorating.

Prints from the 1700s show the practice of sticking holly leaves on window panes (probably with beeswax).

Today we have easy-to-apply adhesives with which to adhere the leaves.

The red berries of holly can be seen to advantage by trimming a few leaves which may obscure the impact of the berries. Or, all the leaves can be trimmed away to leave just berries.

This is a good way to use those stems with poor leaves and great berries.

The stems with berries only can then be used individually in wreaths and arrangements or in clusters.

DECORATING FOR CHRISTMAS WITH HOLLY

The deciduous hollies with long leafless branches of berries are sought after by florists and seen in the swanky hotel lobbies.

They can be purchased if you do not grow them.

Ilex decidua (possumhaw holly) and I. verticillata (winterberry) are often simply sold as "Ilex" in the trade.

ORIENTAL HOLLY

Among the Chinese, Ilex purpurea (synonym Ilex chinensis), the Oriental holly, was much used for decorating temple-courts and large halls during their New Year festivals in February.

For example, Ilex cornuta 'Burfordii' (Chinese holly), with its large clusters of berries, makes a bright red statement, and, for delicate arrangements, I. vomitoria (yaupon holly), with its porcelain berries and neat small leaves, will last several days when cut and placed in water.

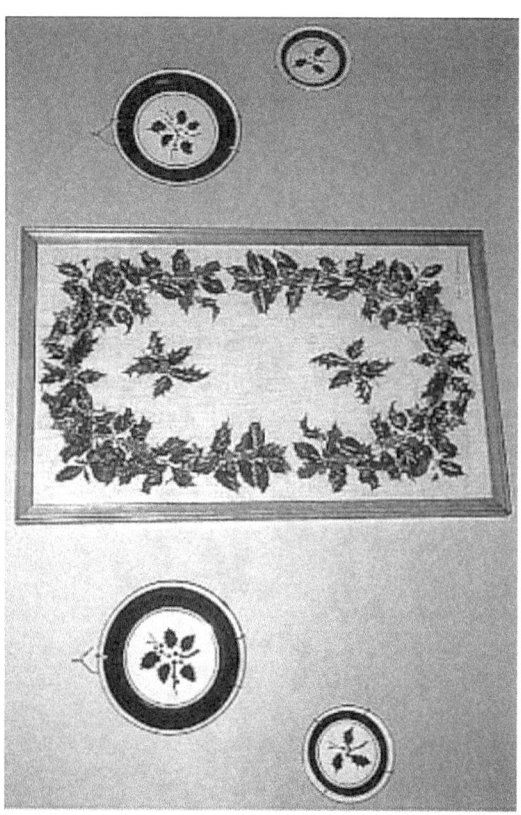

Figure 9. Holly portrait. Photo by Barton Bauer Sr.

GIFT HIDDEN IN SOCKS, U DECORATE TREE MINE,

All the great nations of antiquity, the Assyrians, Egyptians, Persians, Greeks, and Romans decorated their altars, their homes, and their bodies with flowers, and combined leaves and blossoms into wreaths and garlands.

The composition of these floral decorations possessed deep significance and the plants involved had symbolic meaning, being varied according to the social standing of the wearer and the seasons of the year.

In Rome, wreaths of holly were sent newlyweds as tokens of good wishes and congratulations.

CHRISTMAS IN HOLLYWOOD: TOXIC RIDDLE FOR THE TOXIC DETECTIVE

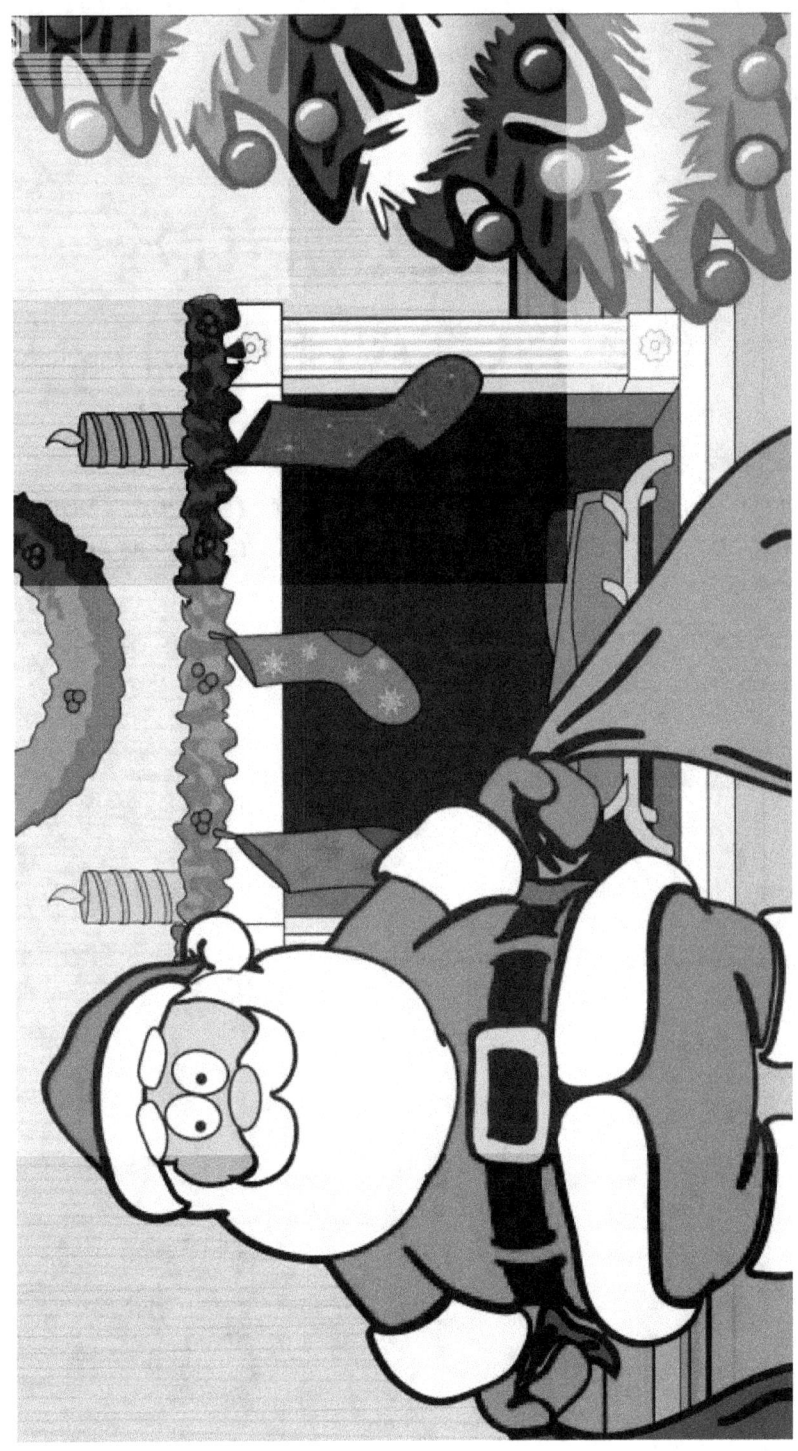

WE DECK UP UR HOUSES AS FRESH AS YOU SAY

Stowe in his *Survey of London* (1598) wrote that every house, the parish churches, all the street corners, and the market places were decorated with holly at Christmas.

Henry Mayhew estimated that 250,000 bunches of holly were sold in London in 1851.

MERRILY GATHER MASS CROWD ROUND MY TREE

About a Nurse

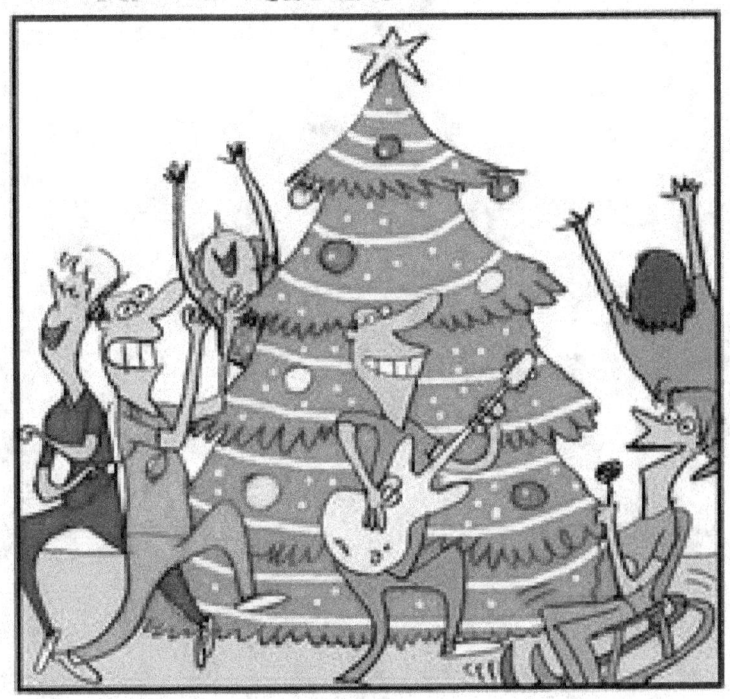

Nurses rocking around the Christmas tree. Have a happy holiday!

Figure 10. Doctors & Nurses celebrate Xmas in Hospitals by merrily gather & crowd around artificial Christmas tree. Image source: **www.allnurses.com**

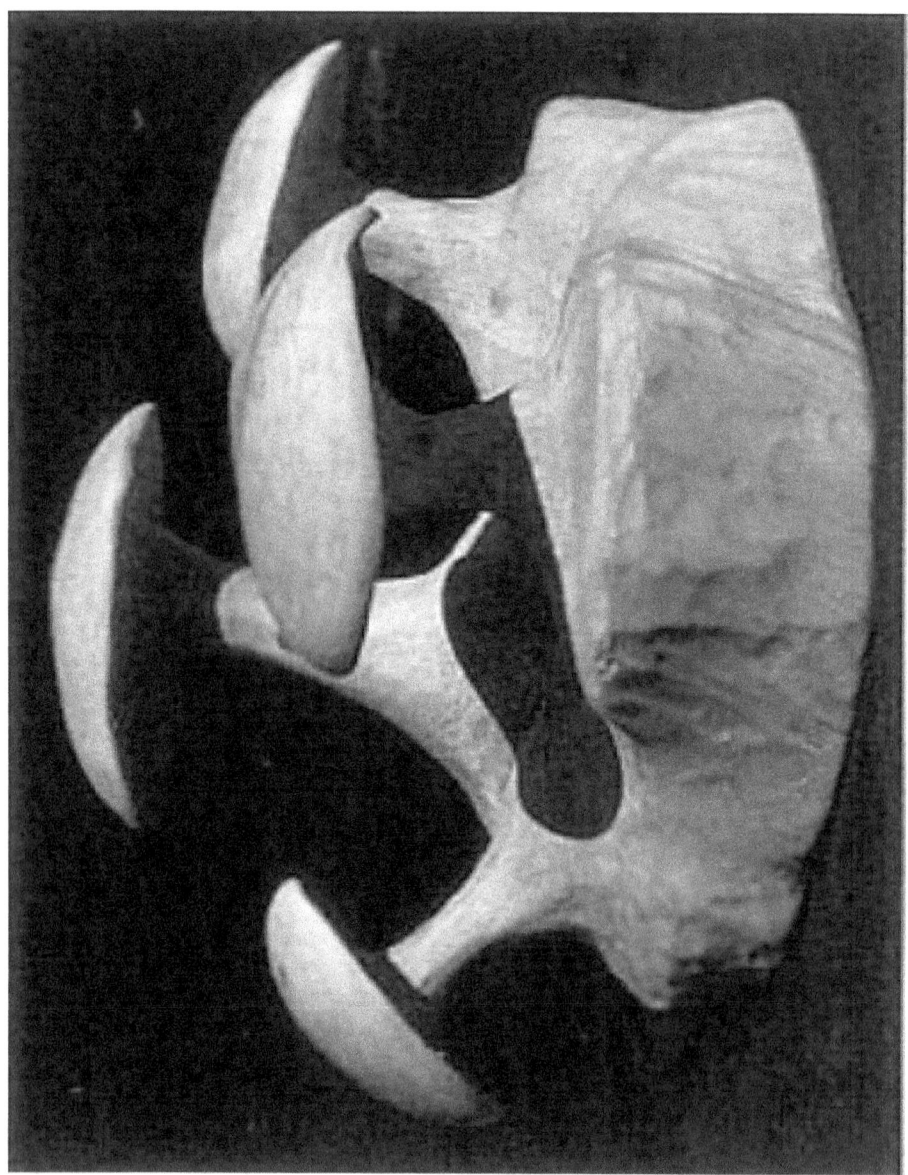

Figure 11. Carving of holly wood. Photo by Fred Galle.

HOLLY WOOD CABINET WORK, TO WHIP-HANDLE

Thus Holly-wood is related to Holly tree, found in USA, to celebrate Christmas, by decorating it.

In the floral vocabulary of the ancients, holly symbolized "defense" and, strangely enough, eastern North American Indians planted holly about their cabins as "protectors," feeling that the trees kept away the evil spirits.

With fruit colored orange, yellow, black, and white in addition to the familiar red, sometimes lasting six months or more, hollies are ideal ornamentals.

Hollies represents years of research by one of the giants of American horticulture, covering all the hollies in cultivation with descriptions of many of the 30 deciduous and 780 evergreen species, including upright trees of 60 feet to creeping prostrate forms.

Fred C. Galle, Holly Society of America Hollies: the genus Ilex. Timber Press.1997.

I OFTEN DISPLAY "A" PYRAMIDAL SPIKE SPREE

Wayside Christmas tree, which has poisonous berries with toxic tannins (tan-in)- cone shaped arrowheads were dipped to hunt & kill Snow mountain deers, for procuring Musk.

" A = symbolises like a pyramid shaped Christmas tree

Did you noticed the coincidence that the riddle no. 200 & 201 have common theme.

200th was based on toxin Musk from Snow- deer(which carries Santa Claus slides on with reins- thus rein-deer).

Riddle No. 201 is based on toxin of Christmas tree

ilex opaca decoded as

I- lacks- opaque A

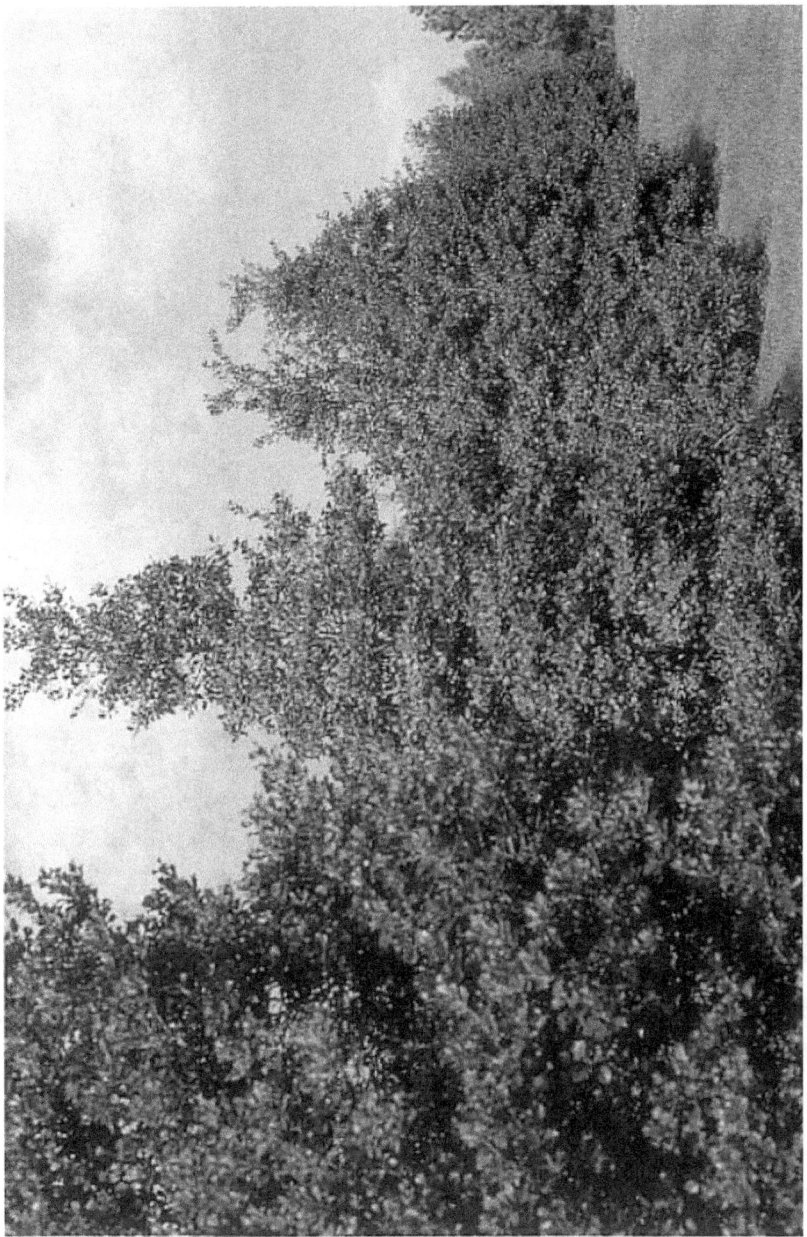

Figure 12. Ilex opaca Pyramidal shape like a cone, at Bernheim Forest Arboretum, Clermont, Kentucky. Photo by Fred Galle.

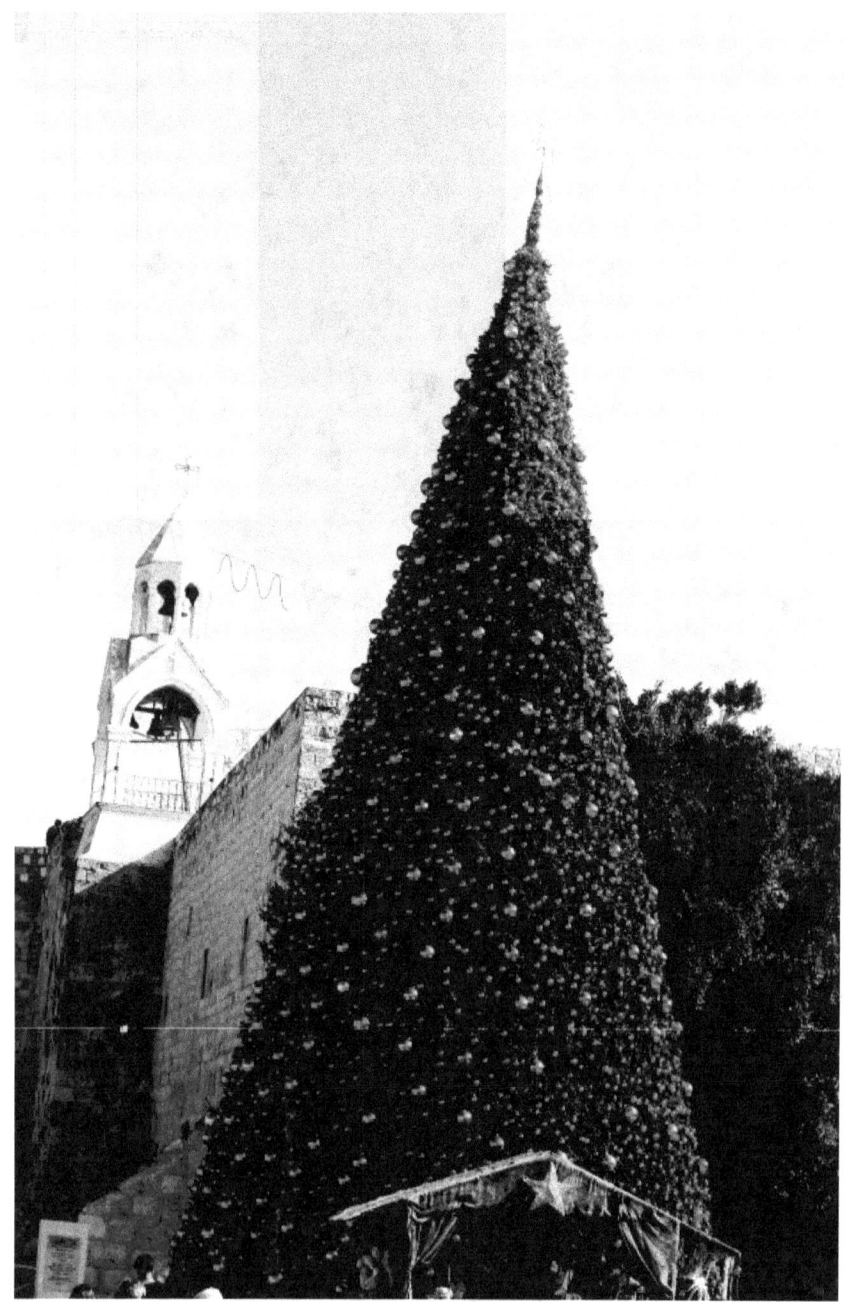

AS THE WHOLLY BRIGHT GIFTS HANG TO DANGLE

In some parts of England, the holly had to be saved until the following year to protect the house from lightning.

In cottages with leaded-pane windows, it was essential that one pane of each window include a sprig of variegated holly in the holiday decorations.

If the Christmas decorations were thrown away, a death in the family would occur before next Christmas. A sprig of holly from church decorations, however, was considered quite valuable and ensured its owner a year of good luck.

Among the early Anglicans of America, holly was kept in their churches until Good Friday to prevent the Christmas festivals from being forgotten.

Berries from the Christmas holly were kept for good luck during the year in Louisiana.

Young branches of holly were cut by the Morbihan peasants in Europe and cured for hay.

The stems were dried, bruised, and fed to cattle three times a day.

Milk and butter from these holly-fed cows were said to be both wholesome and good.

In China the young shoots of Ilex purpurea are sometimes blanched and eaten in salads.

Here, too, the limber twigs of the familiar Chinese holly, I. cornuta, are used as nose rings for cattle.

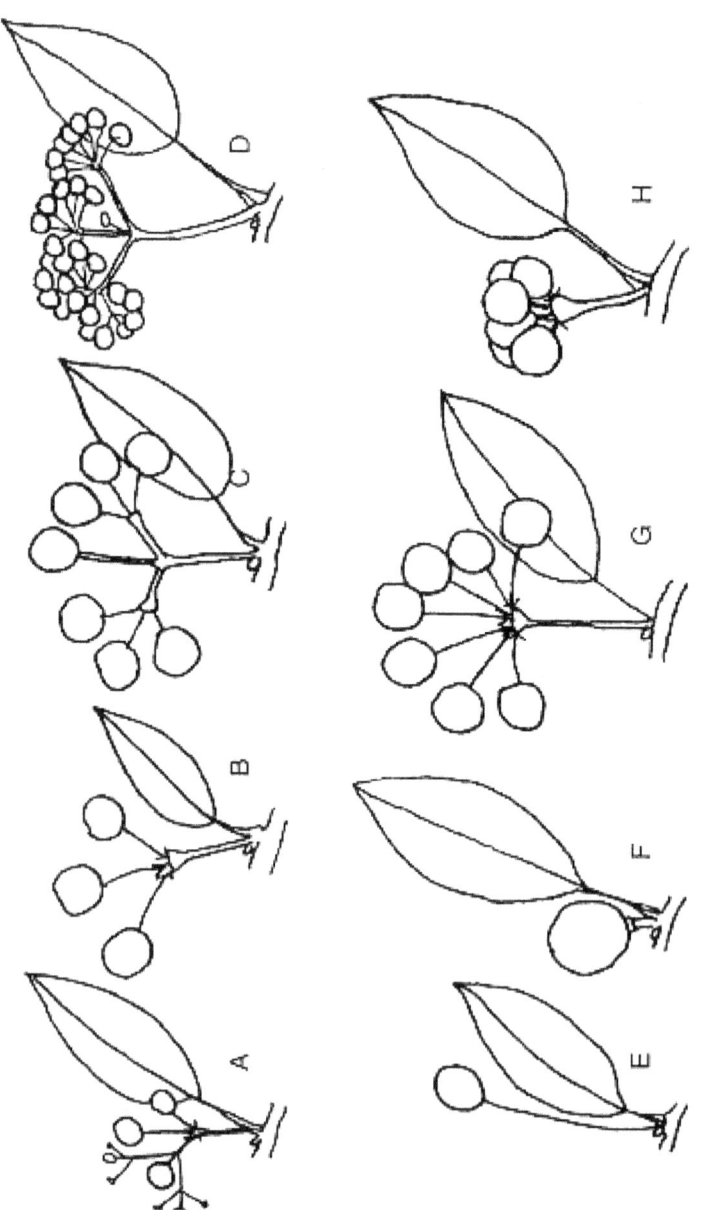

Types of solitary inflorescences in *Ilex*. A, B: simple cymes; C: dichotomous compound cyme; D: trichotomous compound cyme; E: long-pedunculate solitary flower; F: short-pedicellate solitary flower; G: pseudo-umbel; H: headlike inflorescence.

Figure 13. Holly flower pattern

ILEX FLOWERS

More than 80 percent of the Ilex flowers are whitish, pale yellow, or pale greenish yellow; the others are pink to various shades of red to purplish pink.

The flowers of I. intricata are brownish. The pistillate flowers of I. lancilimba are purplish pink and the staminate flowers greenish yellow.

The color of flowers may vary with the habitat of the plant and age of the flowers.

Ilex yunnanensis flowers have been reported as greenish yellow, yellowish white, pink to reddish pink.

There appears to be some correlation of flower color with other characters of the various groups.

All the species in the deciduous-leaved subgenus Prinos have whitish flowers except I. serrata, which has white to reddish pink flowers.

Other sections may be based on flowers that are greenish white to yellowish white or pink to purplish pink. Ilex aquifolium has purplish streaks.

Flowering specimens in herbaria are poorly represented and collection notes on flower color is generally lacking. Flower colors of named cultivars is generally lacking.

The fragrance of Ilex flowers is also often overlooked and not recorded.

This feature should be noted and recorded for all species.

The light fragrance is best observed in early morning and is very attractive to bees.

Ilex latifolia and I. aquifolium are noted for their fragrance.

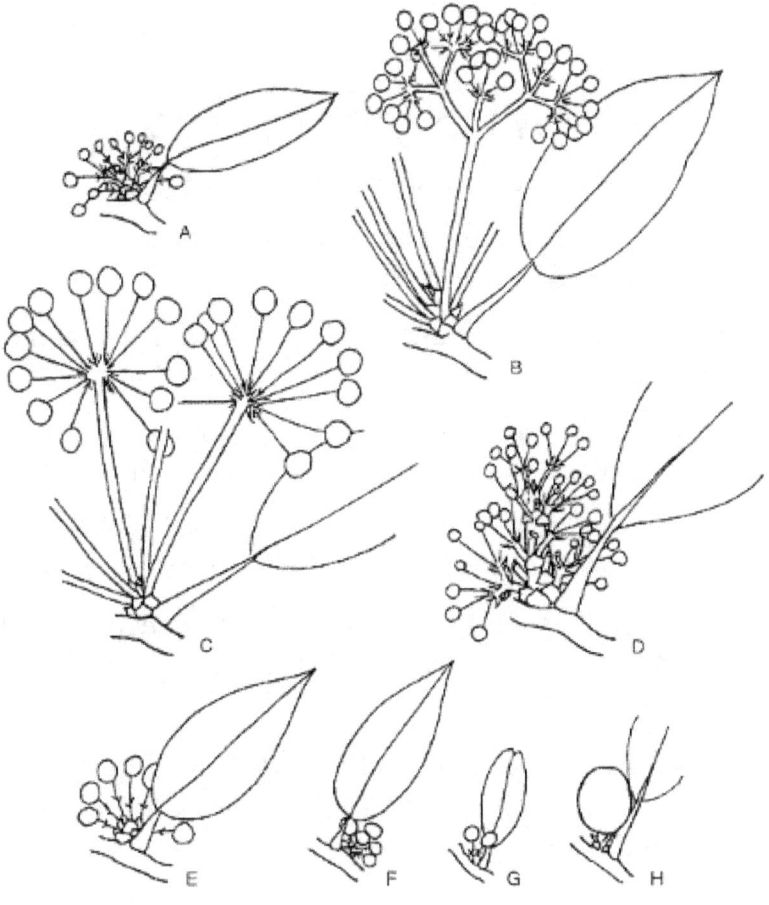

Types of fasciculate inflorescences in *Ilex*. A: fascicle with 1- to 3-flowered individual branches; B: fasciculate compound cymes; C: fasciculate pseudo-umbels; D: pseudopanicle; E: loose fascicle with uniflorous individual branches; F: compact fascicle with uniflorous individual branches; G: paired fruits; H: solitary fruit of a much reduced fascicle.

Figure 14. Ilex Flower buds

FRUITS OF HOLLY

More than 80 percent of Ilex species have red fruit.

S.-y. Hu reported that more than 95 percent of the Chinese Ilex species have red fruits.

Many species from South America have black fruits, and a large number of species have no fruit color recorded.

The fruit matures in autumn and persists for a long time, unless eaten by birds or animals, or until spring when the plant flowers again.

Some species often hold the fruit until the second season.

Red-fruited female species and cultivars are generally esthetically preferred for their attractive displays of fall fruit and are a striking sight in the landscape.

They attract botanist attention for herbarium specimens, but many specimens are only collected in the spring or summer when the fruit is not mature.

CHRISTMAS IN HOLLYWOOD: TOXIC RIDDLE FOR THE TOXIC DETECTIVE

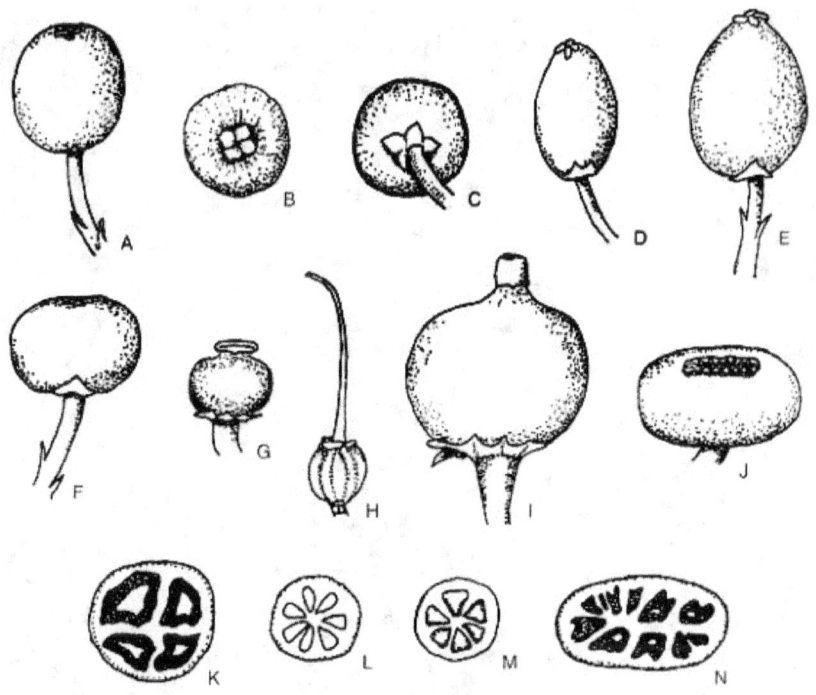

Fruit of *Ilex*. A: lateral view of single fruit of *I. aquifolium*; B: apical view of *I. aquifolium* showing 4 lobed disc-shaped stigma; C: basal view of *I. aquifolium* showing the quadrangular persistent calyx; D: ellipsoid fruit of *I. purpurea*; E: ovoid fruit of a form of *I. opaca* with prophylla on the pedicel; F: compressed-globose or pomiform fruit of *I. opaca*; G: subglobose fruit of *I. fragilis*; H: pendant fruit of *I. asprella* with elongate pedicel, ciliate calyx, and capitate stigma; I: large globose fruit of *I. macrocarpa*; J: compressed subglobose fruit of *I. anomala* with very short pedicel and navel-like stigma; K: cross section of *I. aquifolium* fruit, 4 carpellate, thick-walled endocarps; L: cross section of *I. glabra* fruit, 7 thin-walled endocarps; M: cross section of *I. verticillata* fruit, 6 thin-walled triangular endocarps; N: cross section of *I. anomala* fruit, 11 endocarps, 4 seeded and 7 empty.
Redrawn by Randy Allen from Hume (1959).

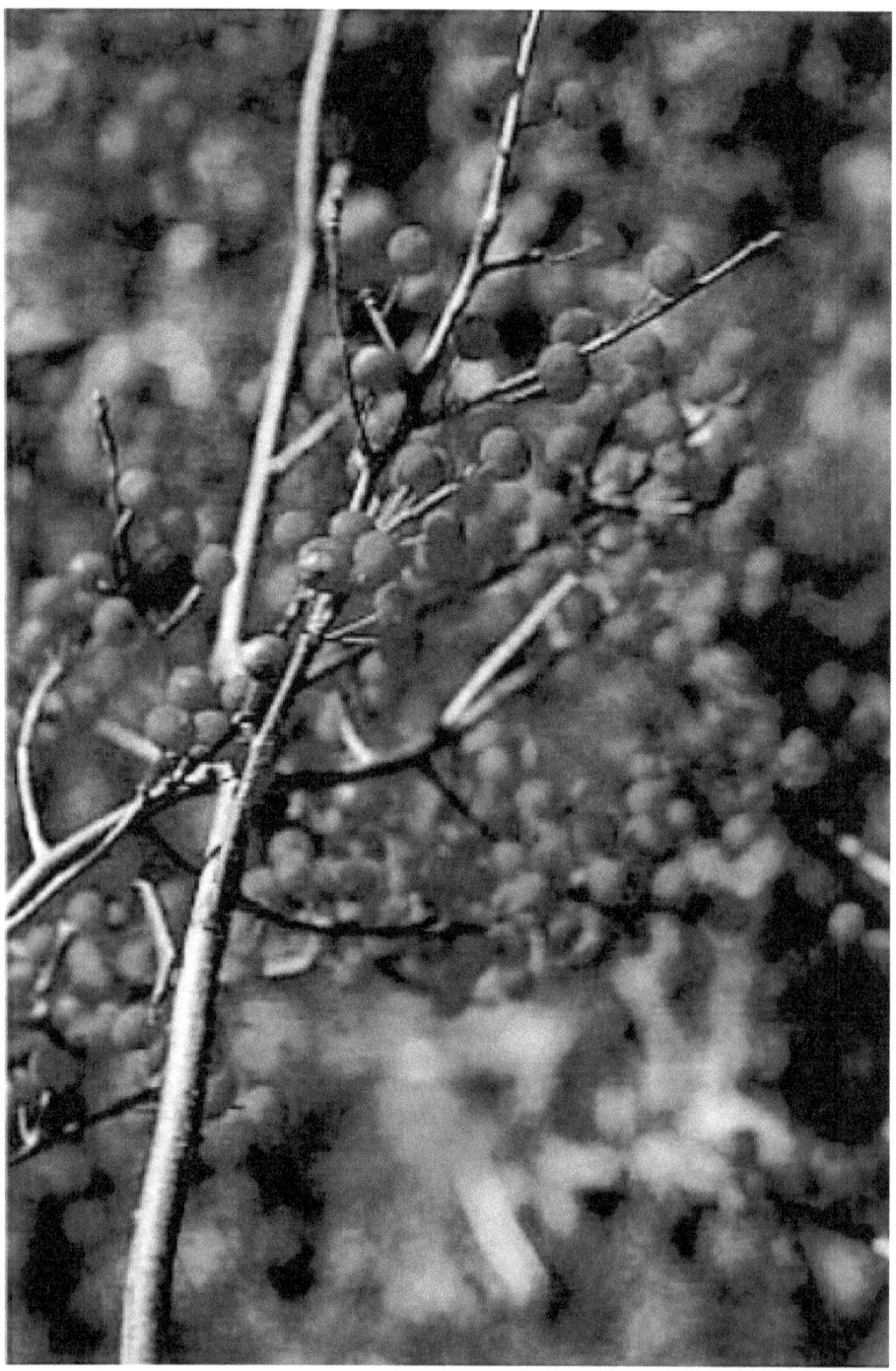

Figure 15. Red Berries of Ilex amelanchier. Photo by Fred Galle.

PEEPS THROUGH TREES WITH BERRIES OF RED,

In a botanical sense, the fruit of Ilex is not a berry nor is it a true drupe, though it is sometimes called a multiseeded drupe or bacco-drupe.

All members of the genus have fleshy fruits (bacco-drupes), chartaceous exocarps, fleshy and often juicy mesocarps, distinct coriaceous, and woody or stony endocarps (pyrenes).

Each endocarp contains a pyrene which in turn contains a seed coat and seed. There is no single term for this type of fruit. In horticulture, a holly fruit is called a berry or a drupe. In 1825 De Candolle used the word bacca (berry).

Later in 1862 Bentham and Hooker used the word drupa (drupe), as did Loesener in the early 1900s.

The holly fruit might be called a drupelike berry or a berrylike drupe.

In 1950 S.Y. Hu proposed the term bacco-drupe, which she defined as a fruit derived from a syncarpous ovary with chartaceous exocarp, fleshy mesocarp, and separated coriaceous, woody or stony endocarps (pyrenes) each containing a single seed.

It is hoped that this term will be accepted in popular usage and in technical literature.

The fruit of Ilex develops from a superior ovary of a compound pistil. It is composed of two or more segments or carpels, usually four with one seed per carpel.

The ovaries of Ilex aquifolium, *I. cornuta*, and *I. opaca* are usually four-carpellate.

As an ovary develops into a mature fruit, the outer layer of cells becomes the exocarp or epidermis and turns red, purplish black, or rarely yellow.

The middle layers of cells, the mesocarp, are a uniform mixture of yellowish or bluish black flesh.

A fleshy mesocarp is described as carnose, a mealy mesocarp as farinose-carnose, and a juicy mesocarp as succose-carnose. The inner layers of cells, the endocarp, develop into separate leathery (coriaceous), or woody (ligneous), or stony compartments. All these tissues are of maternal origin. Each endocarp (pyrene) has a locule containing a single seed.

LEGEND OF RED BERRIES

Legend has it in Brittany that when Christ was bearing His cross, a small bird attempted to relieve His sufferings by plucking thorns from His brow.

The bird's breast became stained with blood and became known forever afterwards as robin redbreast.

To this very day in England and Germany, it is considered unlucky to step on a holly berry, a favorite food of the robin, in recognition of the bird's charitable act.

Native Americans of Pennsylvania regarded the holly as their "Red Badge of Courage" and the token of success in battle.

They knew how to preserve and harden the berries without shrinkage or loss of the brilliant colors.

The preserved berries were used as decorative buttons on vests, sleeves, trousers, and in their hair.

Brisk trading in the berries occurred with tribes where holly did not grow naturally.

PYRENES OF HOLLY

The endocarp containing the seed of Ilex is called the pyrene.

All Ilex pyrenes occur in one whorl embedded in a soft mesocarp.

The abaxial surface or dorsal surfaces are much broader than the lateral or keeled adaxial surface.

About 70 percent of Ilex species have four pyrenes.

CHEMICAL PROPERTIES

The natural chemical properties of Ilex species are seldom discussed in horticultural literature. A review is available in an article by F. Alikarides (1987) of the School of Medicine at the University of Athens, Greece.

The following constituents are described: phenols and phenolic acid, phenyl propanoids, anthocyanins, flavones, terpenoids, sterols, purine alkaloids, amino acids, miscellaneous nitrogen compounds, fatty acids, alkanes and alcohols, carbohydrates, and vitamins and carotenoids.

General and medicinal uses are discussed by Alikarides, followed by a large (154 sources) review of literature.

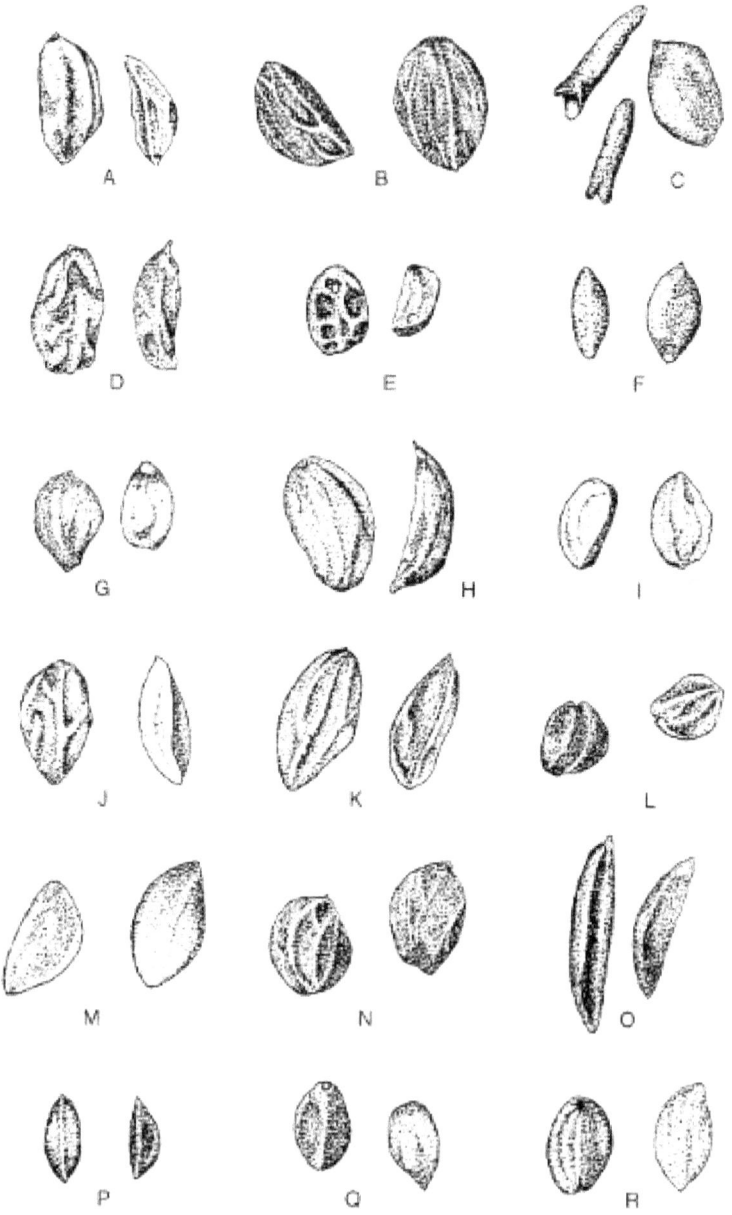

Pyrenes of *Ilex*. A: *I. aquifolium*; B: *I. bioritzensis*; C: *I. coriacea*; D: *I. cornuta*; E: *I. latifolia*; F: *I. laevigata*; G: *I. longipes*; H: *I. macrocarpa*; I: *I. myrtifolia*; J: *I. opaca* 'Cumberland'; K: *I. opaca* 'Miss Helen'; L: *I. paraguariensis*; M: *I. pedunculosa*; N: *I. pernyi*; O: *I. purpurea*; P: *I. rotunda*; Q: *I. serrata*; R: *I. vomitoria*.
Drawing by Randy Allen.

CHRISTMAS IN HOLLYWOOD: TOXIC RIDDLE FOR THE TOXIC DETECTIVE

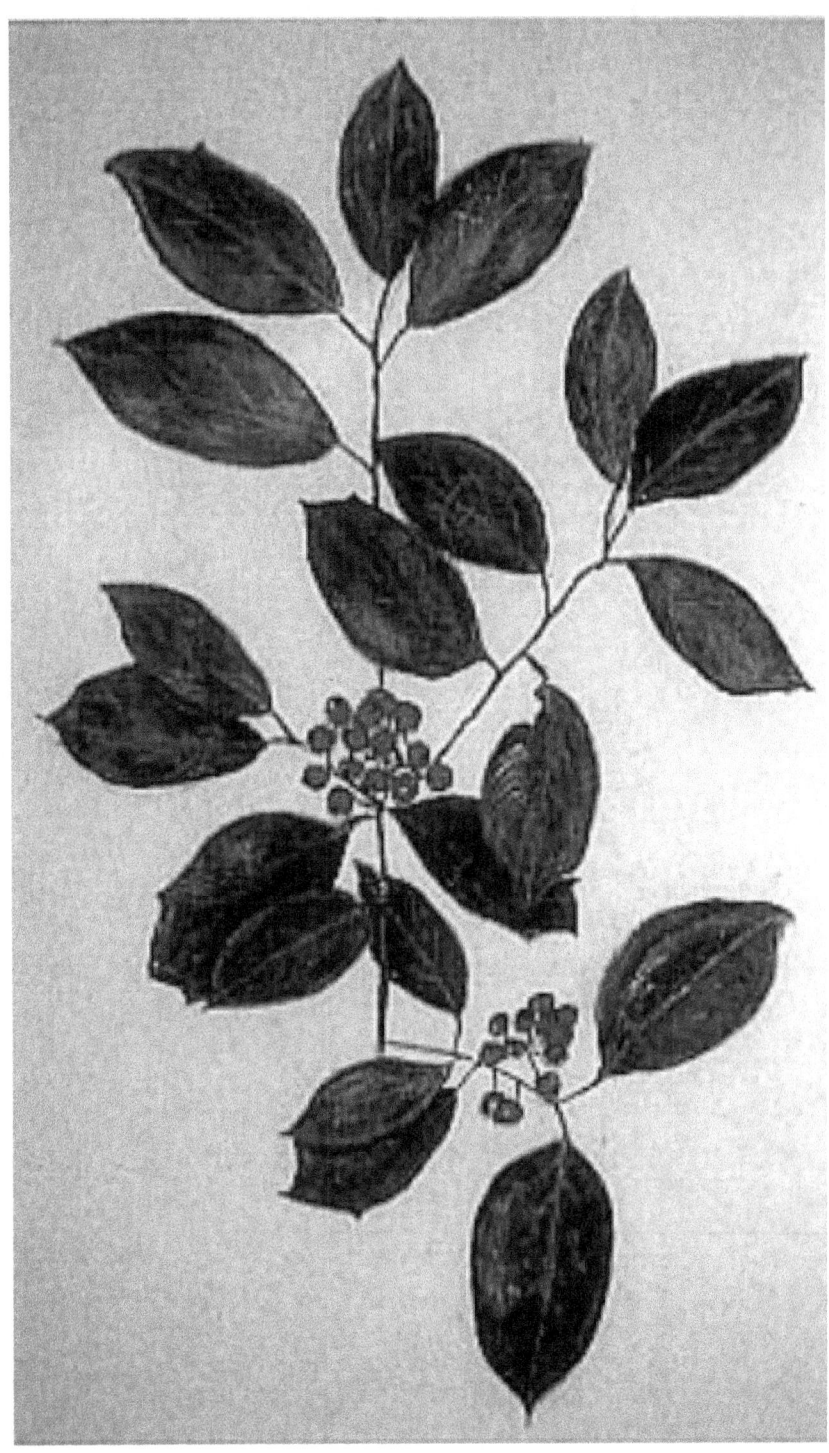

Figure 16. Holly portrait by Peggy Scoggin, 1964. Photo by Fred Galle.

LEAVES OF BURNISHED GREEN SPIKED ANGLE,

A haemolytic principle has been isolated from the leaves (Balansard and Flandrin, 1951).

However, no haemolysis has been reported in human poisoning.

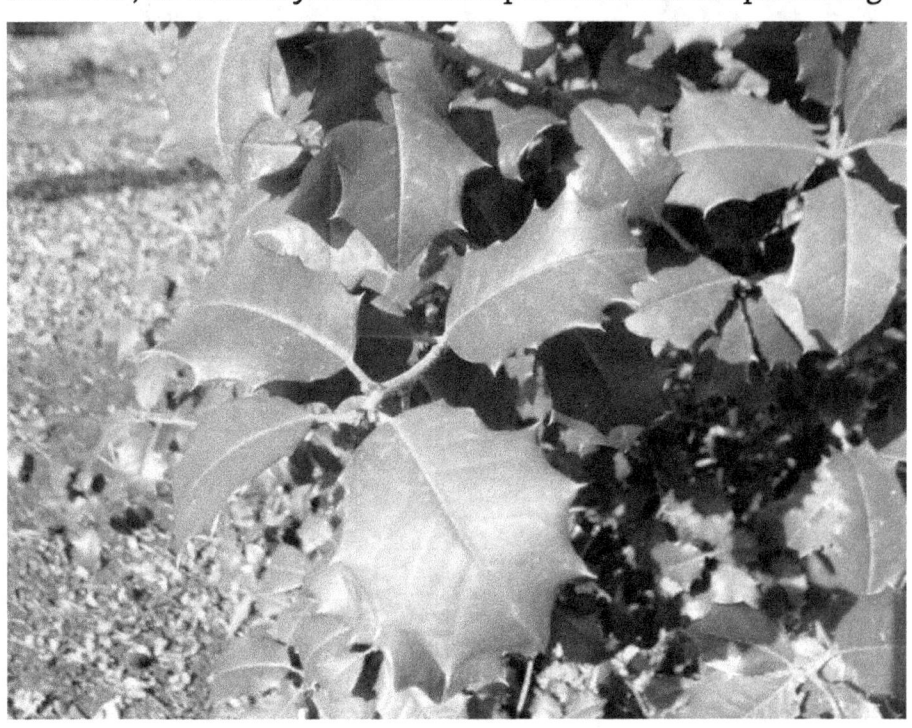

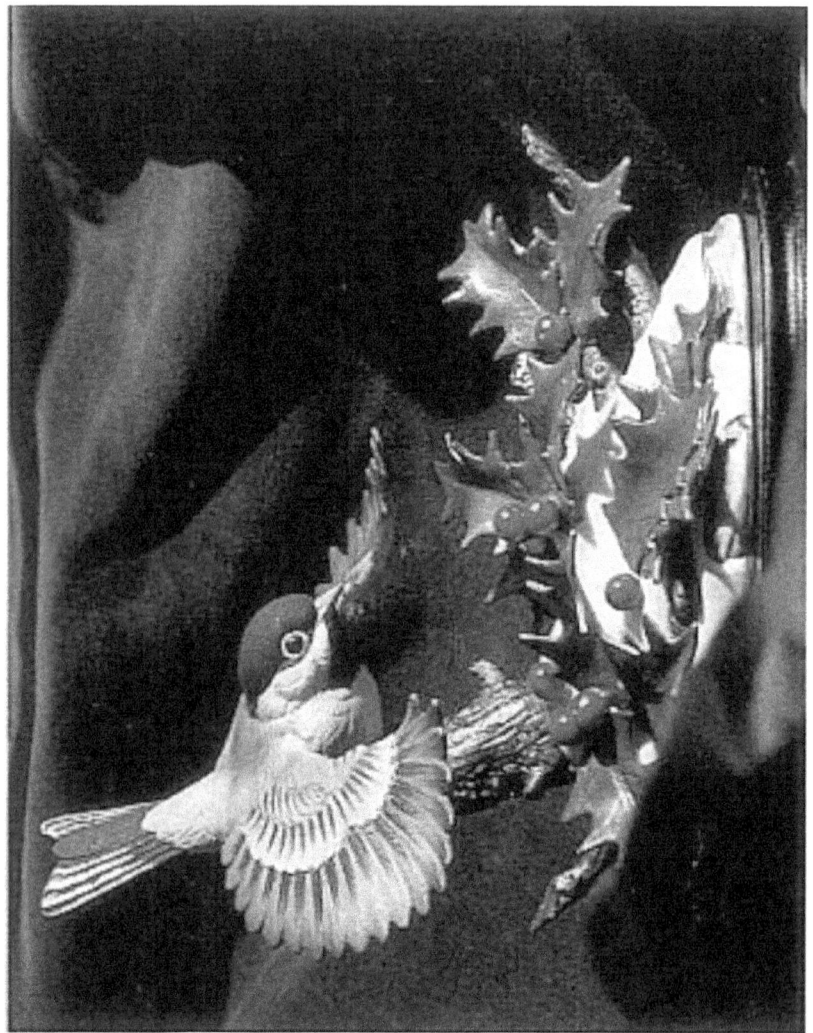

Figure 17. Green Spiky Leaves & Red berries of Holly. Hand-painted holly china. Photo by Barton Bauer Sr.

Mechanical damage to the eye may occur due to the thorny leaves.

The holly, like other thorny plants, was believed in early Europe to repel all evil spirits.

In its name, the witches perceived the word holy, and its spiny foliage and blood-red berries were suggestive of Christian associations.

Pliny the Elder wrote that a holly tree planted about the house served as a counter-charm and kept away all evil spirits or enchantments and defended the house from lightning.

Branches of holly were hung about the homes and stables, and cattle were said to thrive if a piece of holly was hung where it could be seen on Christmas Day.

Canes of holly were formerly highly prized in early England.

Fast-growing, young shoots of holly made excellent walking sticks and were carried by maidens and matrons alike as protection against mad dogs, vicious beasts, and other perils of the day.

As early as 507 B.C. Pythagoras wrote that if a staff made of holly is flung at a (mad) dog, the beast would lie quietly near it.

Henry Phillips in 1823, however, deemed quite credulous the old customs of his ancestors, who trusted branches of holly to defend them against witchcraft.

"But this precaution," he wrote, "has become unnecessary, since old ladies have lost their charming powers, and the spells of the youthful fair are too agreeable to be driven from us by a rod of holly."

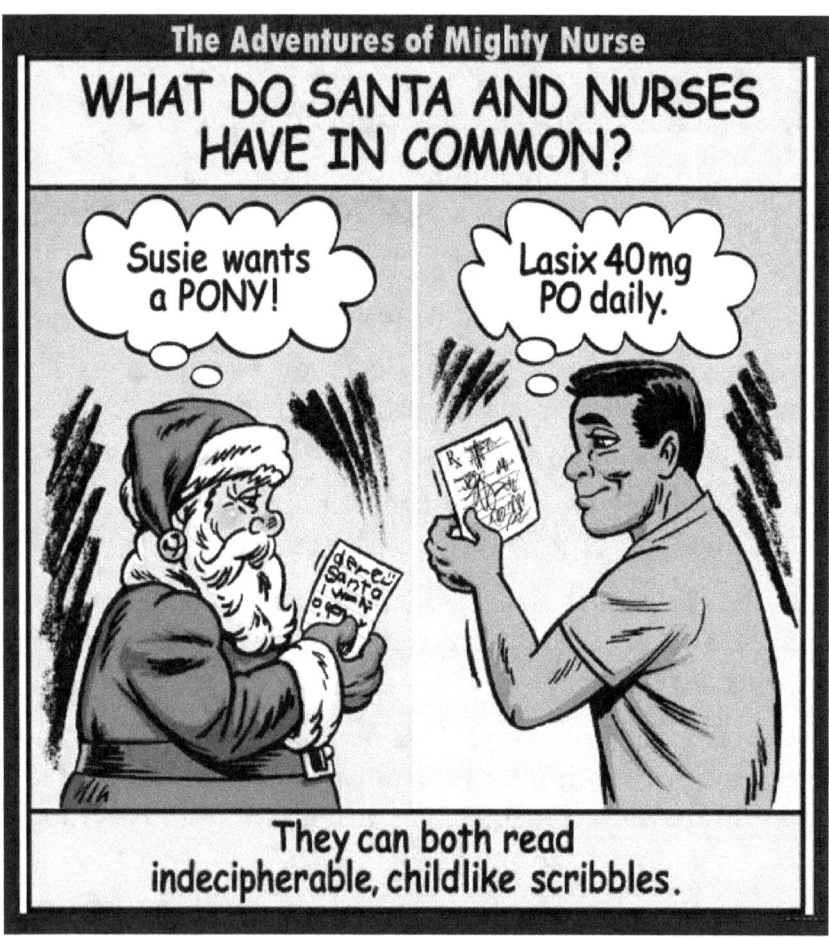

Figure 18. Deciphering scrabble- Analogy between santa & Nurse. Image source: www.mightynurse.com

HOLLY'S HERBAL TEA

In more modern times, infusions, decoctions, and fomentations of holly were used for a wide assortment of human disorders.

In England, a tea of holly bark was a cure for the cough.

In France, a decoction of leaves and bark was considered equal to and sometimes better than quinine in the treatment of intermittent fever.

A tea of holly leaves was a cure for measles by some North American Indian tribes, while an elixir of the leaves, bark, and wood was regarded by them as a specific against disease.

A beverage of the berries pacified Cherokee women and curbed their urge for wandering.

The juice of holly leaves was also good for pain in the side.

Native American women wore sprigs of holly during childbirth, believing them to ease the pain and to ensure the delivery of healthy offspring.

CHINESE HOLLY

It is interesting to note that the leaves of one holly frequently used for tea by people living on the Chinese-Tibetan border come from Ilex yunnanensis var. eciliate, which is related to I. vomitoria and has been used in a similar way as the hollies used by tribal groups in both North and South America since ancient times.

HOLLY & WHOLLY

John Evelyn, in 1662, related that a posset made of milk and beer in which the most pointed holly leaves are boiled is certain to abate torments of colic when all else failed.

Leaves of holly, he reported, when dried to a fine powder and drunk in white wine prevail against gall stones.

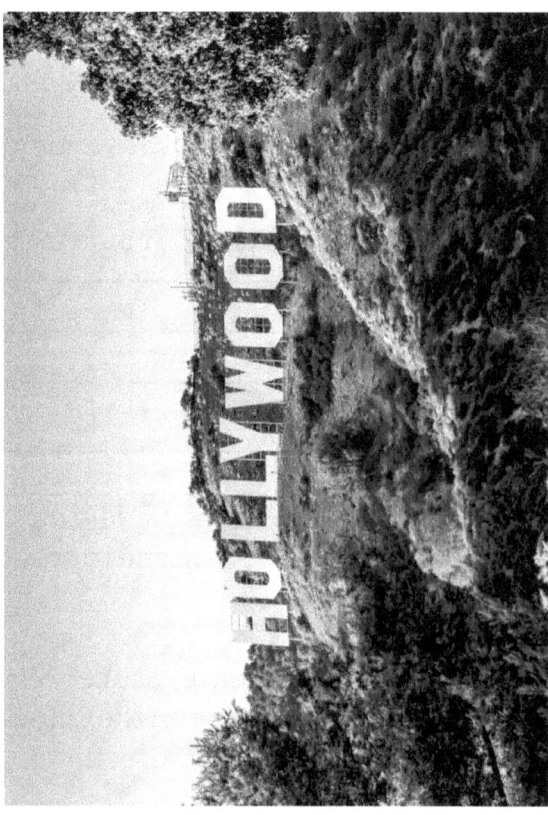

Figure 19. Hollywood, the cinema site of USA

HOLLYWOOD- WHAT'S IN NAME

Hollywood, is the cinematic site of USA, where maximum Oscar award winning movies had been shot.

The name Hollywood might originated from the shooting stage in 1900's prepared from woods derived from Holly plant species, as plastics was discovered yet, and timber wood was used to set up the artificial stages to recreate the scene.

Bollywood name was derived from Hollywood, which means the Bombay cinema studios located in Mumbai.

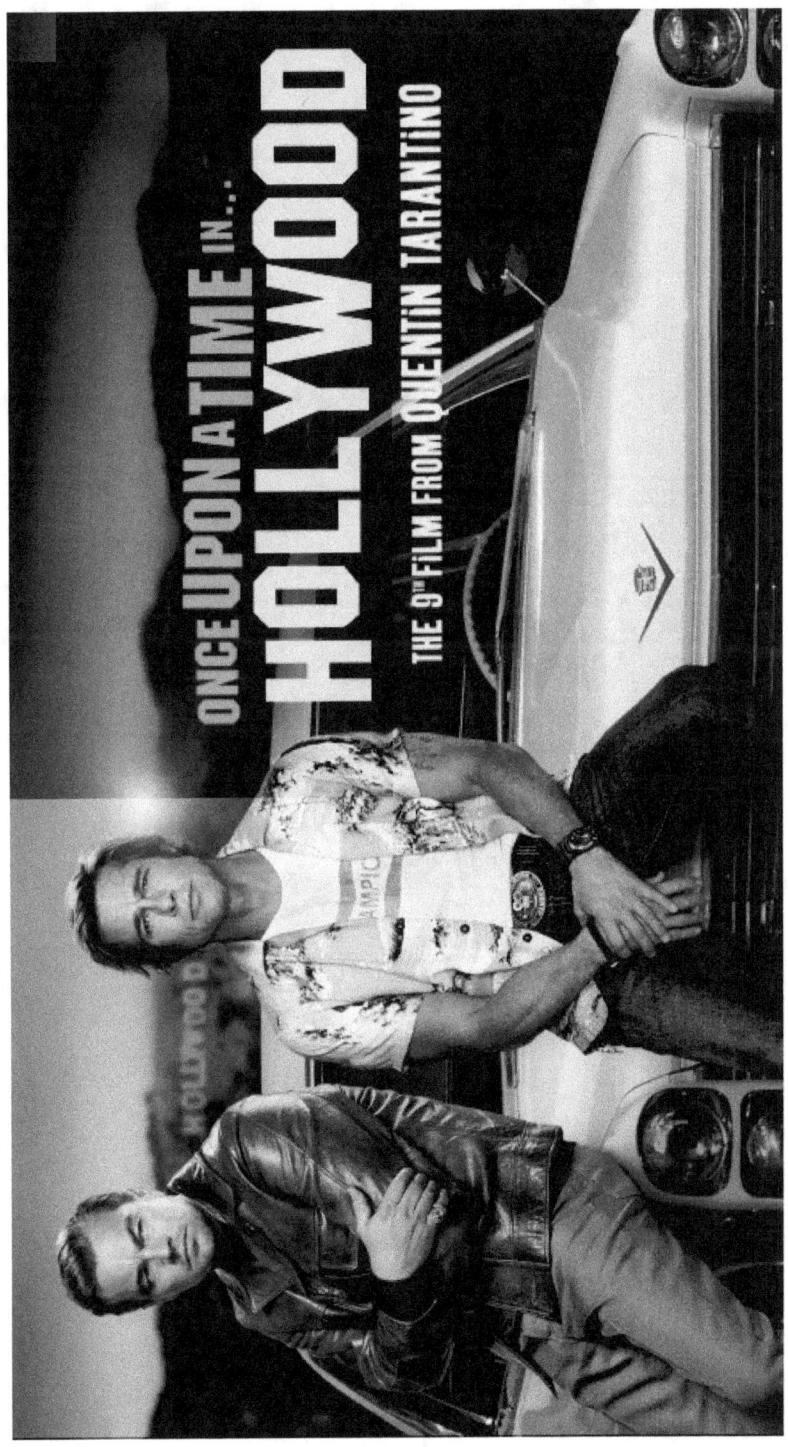

Figure 20. Once upon a time in Hollywood (2019) Movie

HOLLY WOOD'S CUP DRINKS CURED TOTALLY

In England, an old cure for chilblains was to thrash them soundly with branches of holly; a rustic specific for whooping cough was to drink new milk out of a cup made from the wood of variegated holly.

Followers of Zoroaster in Persia and India used an infusion of water and holly bark to sprinkle the faces of newborn children.

JOLLY'S TOOTHACHE CURED BY HOLLY

An old and quaint English cure for toothache concerns the belief that the pain was caused by the gnawing of little worms inside the tooth.

The remedy for this was to hold a smoldering holly coal in the mouth so that the smoke could enter the cavity of the afflicted part.

This promptly dispatched the tiny offenders and caused them to drop out of the tooth.

While all these remedies have been attributed to our familiar American and English Christmas hollies, other members of this same family have likewise contributed to the well-being of the world.

BARK TO DISINFECT

In the far East, decoctions of the bark and leafy shoots of the familiar Chinese holly, Ilex cornuta, are commonly used as tonics, especially for the kidneys; the crushed seeds of this species are frequently used in medicines.

Among the people of the Saint Helena Islands of South Carolina, a mixture of lard and Ilex cassine, mockingbird bush, is used as an ointment for smallpox.

Farther northward, the berries and bark of Ilex verticillata, winterberry, the deciduous holly, have often been substituted for Peruvian bark in cases of intermittent fevers.

The bark has also been used as a wash for gangrene and eruptions of the skin.

Ilex cassine, the dahoon holly, was used by the early settlers of North Carolina to purify the coastal swamp water and render it fit to drink.

Waud RA (1932). Further studies on extracts made from holly. Proc Soc Exp Biol Med 30: 393-398.

HOLLIES

European Holly, English Holly, Oregon Holly, Sparked Holly, Christmas Holly, Crocodile Holly, Prick Holly, Holly, Common Holly, Holly Green.

MY ATTRACTIVE FRUITS ARE HARMFUL, AS I SAID

Poisoning by ilex is due to the ingestion of berries, which may induce gastrointestinal symptoms.

Ingestion of berries may cause nausea, vomiting, abdominal pain and diarrhoea.

Stupor and drowsiness have been seen in children after ingestion of large quantities of berries. Although lethal cases have been reported in older literature there are no recent reports of severe poisonings.

Intoxications are almost exclusively seen in children after ingestion of berries from Ilex aquifolium cultivated in parks, gardens, or when branches with berries are used ornamentally in homes.

TOXINS

Several active principles have been identified:

- Phenolic derivatives: vanillic acid, p-hydroxybenzoic acid (fruit); Anthocyanines: cyanidin-3-xylosylglucoside (fruit); pelargonidin-3-glucoside (fruit);

- Flavonoids: quercetin-3-rutinoside (leaves) Terpenoids: alpha-amyrin (bark, leaves, fruit); ursolic acid (leaves, fruit); oleanolic acid (leaves); ilex lactone (fruit); Sterols: ergosterol (leaves); beta-sitosterol (fruit); Alkaloids: theobromine, Fatty acids: pentadecanoic acid (leaves); palmitic acid (leaves); stearic acid (leaves); arachidic acid (leaves); oleic acid (leaves); linolenic acid (leaves); Alkanes: (leaves, fruit)

- Cyanogenic glucosides: 2 beta-D-glucopyranosyloxy-p-hydroxy-6,7-dihydromandelonitrile (fruit, leaves, bark).

- Ilex lactone: 3-(3'-Hydroxycyclopent-1-enyl-Z-propenicacid-1,5'-lactone

- Triterpenester: 27,p-cumaroxy ursolic acid.

Citation: Thomas H, Budzikiewicz H (1980). Ilex lactone, ein bis-normonoterpen neuartiger strukture aus Ilex aquifolium. Phytochemistry 19: 1866-1868.

FATAL DOSE

3 - 5 berries may cause gastrointestinal symptoms.

Although 20 to 30 berries are estimated to be a "lethal dose".

Rodriguez TD, Johnson PN, Jeffrey LP (1984). Holly berry ingestion: case report. Vet Hum Toxicol 26: 157-158.

FATAL PERIOD

Gastrointestinal symptoms appear within hours after the ingestion of berries and may last for 24 hours.

Severe symptoms may be observed after ingestion of a large number of berries.

Death has been reported in the older literature (Lewin, 1929), but has not been confirmed by more recent reports.

HOLLY'S MELANCHOLY

Culpeper, in his pithy herbals of 1653, related that holly is governed by the planet Saturn and thus influences the "melancholy," a sediment of the blood whose receptacle was the spleen.

The holly, like other Saturnine plants, was therefore considered "cold and dry in quality, fortifying the retentive faculty, and memory; makes men sober, solid, and staid, fit for study; stays the unbridled joys of lustful blood, stays the wandering thoughts; and reduces them home to the centre."

Writing specifically about the virtues of the holly tree, Culpeper stated that the berries expel wind and are, therefore, good for the colic.

If a dozen ripe berries were eaten in the morning before fasting, they purged the body of wastes.

If, however, the berries were first dried and beaten into a powder, they bound the body and stopped bleeding and fluxes.

The bark of the tree and also the leaves are exceptionally good, being used in fomentations for broken bones and for such members as are out of joint.

Girarde, in his herbal of 1597, some fifty years earlier, had published Culpeper's remedies in language more picturesque than printable.

HOLIDAY PLANTS WITH TOXIC MISCONCEPTIONS

Most ingestions cause little or no toxicity.

The primary clinical effects observed, which occur exclusively with large ingestions, include nausea, vomiting, abdominal cramping, and occasionally dermatitis.

There can be allergic sensitization and worsening dermatitis with repeat exposures.

Rarely, mydriasis, hyperthermia, and drowsiness have also been reported.

Evens ZN, Stellpflug SJ. Holiday plants with toxic misconceptions. West J Emerg Med. 2012;13(6):538-542. doi:10.5811/westjem.2012.8.12572

DIAGNOSIS

There are no specific laboratory analyses.

A sample of the berries and leaves is useful for identification.

Sample of vomitus or gastric lavage fluid may be useful for identification of the berries.

Identification of the plant and berries is easy.

FIRST-AID MEASURES AND MANAGEMENT PRINCIPLES

Emesis or gastric lavage is indicated, especially in children if more than 3-5 berries have been ingested. Treatment is supportive in the symptomatic patient.

Emesis or gastric lavage may be indicated in recent ingestion of more than 5-10 berries in an adult.

Hospitalization is indicated if large amounts have been ingested.

Symptomatic treatment of gastrointestinal symptoms.

Replacement of fluids and electrolyte losses in the case of vomiting and diarrhea.

The Best Medicine

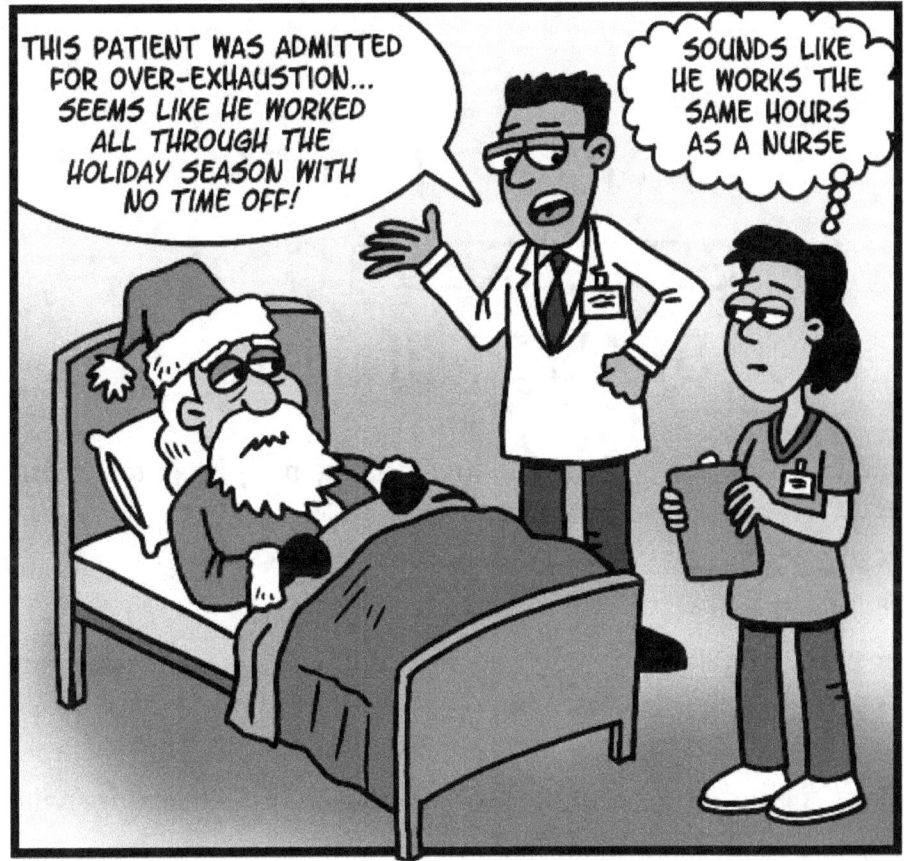

AND SO NEVER GET LURED TO MY BEAUTIFUL HUE,

Many superstitions existed about bringing in the holly for Christmas.

In Wales, if it was brought in before Christmas Eve, it was sure to cause family quarrels throughout the year.

In parts of Germany and England, the prickly varieties were known as he-hollies, while the smooth-leaved kinds were called she-hollies.

The type of holly brought into the household determined who was to dominate the home during the year.

If the holly was smooth, the wife was in command; if the holly was prickly, the husband governed for the year.

This later custom was brought to the New World and was known in the late nineteenth century among the Ulster Scots of Pennsylvania.

Here, the belief existed, too, that if the holly was brought into the house in good weather, the wife would master the household for the ensuing year, but if brought in during rough weather, the husband would be the ruler.

Superstitions, too, existed regarding the removal of the holly after Christmas.

In some parts of England, it was decidedly unlucky to leave holly up after New Year's Eve, or Twelfth Night (6 January, the final day of Christmas celebrations), lest the maidens of the household be visited by a ghost for each leaf in the decorations.

Others said that a misfortune for each leaf would befall those unheeding this rule.

The holly could not merely be thrown away but had to be burnt, else the ill luck would continue as though the holly had not been removed.

> Elsewhere in England, holly had to be taken down before Shrove Tuesday (Mardi Gras, the last day before Lent) and burnt on the same fire on which the pancakes were to be baked; misfortune was to be certain to befall anyone so unwise as not to heed this belief.

WARN UNTO MY TOXIC RED BERRIES, LIKE YEW

Toxic Berries of Hollies are look alike (bright red berries) & act alike (cardiotoxic) Yews.

Of all old English traditions, however, one of the most enchanting is that even the bees must be wished a Merry Christmas: a sprig of shiny green and bright red holly must adorn each hive.

FOR KIDS & PETS
MIGHT ATE TO
MANHANDLE,

TWIN HOLLIES

Rodrigues et al.(), describes a case of 2 identical twins that ingested a "handful" of holly berries.

One twin vomited 40 times over 6 hours and was drowsy, while the other twin had only 5 episodes of emesis in the same time period without drowsiness.

Poisonings most often occur in children, and most cases are harmless.

In adults, one must eat 20-30 berries before becoming symptomatic, whereas children only have to consume five berries to develop toxicity.

Wink M, van Wyk BE. Mind-Altering and Poisonous Plants of the World. Portland: Timber Press, 2008.

IPECAC IN HOLLY

One study attempted to explore management techniques for pediatric ingestions of toxic berries (including holly berries), comparing home observation alone with syrup of ipecac and home observation.

Predictably, all of the patients in the ipecac group vomited, while there was no vomiting among the subjects in the home observation alone group.

There was more sedation and diarrhea in the ipecac group as well.

Wax PM, Cobaugh DJ, Lawrence RA. Should home ipeac-induced emesis be routinely recommended in the management of toxic berry ingestions. Vet Hum Toxicol. 1999;41:394-7

Ipecac is no longer recommended for toxic ingestions in general.

ED therapy recommendations for holly berry exposures include symptomatic management, such as antiemetics, along with fluid and electrolyte supplementation for dehydration from rare severe vomiting and diarrhea.

AS BERRIES ARE FATAL, TURNS CYANOTIC BLUE

The berries containing the toxin saponin are poisonous; the leaves are not.

The toxic component of the berries is saponin.

The primary potential biological effect of saponin is a negative interaction with cellular membranes.

Saponins can cause hemolysis in erythrocytes and alterations in permeability of small intestinal mucosal cells.

IT'S NATURE'S GIFT, TO PROTECT AGAINST VANDAL

Most of the Flowering Trees, protect their fruits by different means, some by synthesizing toxin in fruit pulp, some add toxic alkaloids in the seeds, or built spines or thorns on their stems, or make their coating hard like stone.

Quite apart from the holly superstitions associated with Christmas are those related to divination, the pretended art of foreseeing future events by supernatural or magical means.

Perhaps, to paraphrase Folkard, the most interested in this form of sorcery were those vain and silly maidens who no longer could endure the suspense of not knowing the names of their future husbands.

There had to be three maidens for the magic to work.

Off they would go to the house of the old witch, who would show them how to construct a witch's chain of holly, juniper, and mistletoe berries with an acorn at the end of each link, and how to wind these beads around a slender wand of wood.

This was to be placed on the fire with magical sayings and, as the last acorn was burnt, each would see her future husband walk across the room.

A less expensive but more painful method of seeing a future husband in early England was for the maiden to place three pails of water on her bedroom floor.

Upon retiring, she pinned three leaves of holly on her nightdress, opposite her heart.

During her sleep, she would be awakened by three loud yells, followed by three coarse laughs; after this, the form of her future husband would be seen.

The intensity of his love for the maiden was determined by whether or not the pails were disturbed.

Unfortunately, this charm was only potent if carried out on Halloween, Midsummer Eve, New Year's Eve, and Christmas Eve.

Another traditional form of foreseeing the future in parts of England consisted of collecting nine smooth-leaved (she-holly) leaves and placing them in a three-cornered handkerchief that had to be tied with nine knots.

The knotted handkerchief was placed under the pillow and during sleep, pleasant dreams of the future were certain to ensue.

For this spell to be fully effective the holly leaves had to be picked late on a Friday and the utmost care taken to maintain complete silence until the following morning.

A quaint fortune-telling superstition of England consisted of fixing little candles on holly leaves and placing them in a pan of water.

If the leafy vessels floated, it was a sure sign that the project the person had in mind at the time would prosper.

If, however, they sank, the person would do well to abandon the idea as soon as possible.

Tornio, Stacy. Plants That Can Kill 101 Toxic Species to Make You

Think Twice. 2017

BEVERAGE

Palatable and stimulating is a tealike beverage called "maté," "yerba matá," or "Paraguay tea." Brewed from leaves of *Ilex paraguariensis*, one of several South American hollies, maté is an all purpose drink used by more than thirty million South Americans daily, principally in Paraguay and Argentina.

An early South American Indian custom still practiced today is to serve visitors a gourd of maté.

The chief sips some of the tea through a *bombilla* and passes the receptacle to the visitor, who drinks from the same tube.

Everyone in camp partakes of the beverage until it is consumed.

It is an act of unpardonable rudeness to refuse to drink any of the maté.

Maté is recognized by the chemists as a stimulant for the nerves and muscles as well as for the brain. During World War I, the British, French, and German armies found it to be a valuable stimulant in times of stress.

High in the eastern side of Ecuador's Andes, the Zapara and Jibaro Indians have used *guayusa* since pre-Columbian times.

This tea is brewed from another South American holly, *Ilex guayusa*, related to but distinct from *I. paraguariensis*.

In appearance *I. guayusa* is not unlike the old holly trees of England.

EMETIC

While quite acceptable as a substitute for coffee or tea, the infusion, as brewed by these Indians, is so strong that it acts as an emetic.

The *guayusa* pot is kept carefully covered and the brew simmered over a slow fire throughout the night. On rising in the morning, the Indians would drink enough to make them vomit, believing that the beverage conferred strength and swiftness to the hunter.

Groves of this holly were planted about the villages of the Indians.

BLACK DRINK

Since ancient times Native Americans in what became southern United States held in greatest esteem the celebrated "black drink" or "cassena," brewed from the toasted leaves of *Ilex vomitoria,* the yaupon of southeastern United States.

This holly tea restored lost appetites, confirmed health, and gave its drinkers courage and agility in war.

Accounts of the black drink ceremony were recorded as long ago as 1536.

Participants in the ceremony gathered in the spring of the year, along the sea coast where the yaupon grew in abundance, some traveling several hundred miles to attend the rituals.

The holly leaves were parched in earthenware vessels over fires and then boiled for a considerable period.

While the leaves were brewing, the pot was kept carefully covered, but if by chance any women came into the vicinity while the pot was uncovered, the men threw the drink away, believing that some evil would be imparted to the beverage.

No woman was allowed to move or walk about during the cooling and serving process and should, perchance, this occur, the men would throw the drink away, disgorge what they had already swallowed, and severely punish the transgressing female.

At the same time, the men continually called out, "Who will drink?" Who will drink?" Any woman within hearing distance of the shouts was obliged to remain motionless, even if standing on tiptoes, until the men had consumed their fill.

> On other occasions, the cassine was used in ceremonies concerned with the well-being of the tribe. Sitting at the head of a semicircular bench, the chief, with his councilors and elders, accepted the blessing of those who were to partake of the drink. Having accepted a salutation from each brave starting with the eldest, the chief ordered the women to brew the drink.

> Matters of importance to the tribe were discussed and debated by the priests, elders, and nobles of the tribe. No decisions were made until a number of councils had carefully deliberated the opinions and recommendations of the

speakers.

During the discussions, the chief was served the hot drink in a capacious shell.

The chief, in turn, directed the rest to drink from the same vessel.

ORDEAL POISON to TEST

So esteemed did Native Americans hold this holly tea that no one was allowed to drink it during the council except those proved to be brave and courageous warriors.

So strong was this beverage that it immediately threw the drinker into a deep sweat.

Those whose stomachs rejected the beverage were not to be trusted to any difficult or warlike mission.

The drink was believed to nourish and strengthen the body. Some sixty species of hollies yield leaves for beverage purposes.

Its use in Americans tribals just like African tribal people of Old Calabar used Calabar beans or 'E-ser-e' as an ordeal poison, and administered them to persons accused of witchcraft or other crimes. It was considered to affect only the guilty; if a person accused of a crime ingested the beans without dying, they were considered innocent.

Goldfrank's toxicologic emergencies. Hoffman, Robert S. (Robert Steven), 1959-, Howland, Mary Ann,, Lewin, Neal A.,, Nelson, Lewis, 1963-, Goldfrank, Lewis R., 1941-, Flomenbaum, Neal (Tenth ed.). New York. 2014-12-23

AS BERRIES CAUSES CARDIAC ARREST, IF ADDED TO BREW

Despite these varied and valued healing properties of holly and its contributions to the medicinal lore of the Old World, it is of interest to note two old Welsh superstitions: to pluck a sprig of holly in flower was a sure cause of death in the family of the picker, and holly must never be brought into a sick room for the patient was almost surely to suffer a relapse or die as a consequence.

The experiments were undertaken by Dr Waud Russell A., et al (1931) in the Department of Pharmacology, University of Western Ontario Medical School, London, Canada to determine the effects of extracts of the above Ilex fruit on the amphibian heart, Male frogs (Ram pipiens) were used.

Citation: Waud, R. A. Action of Ilex Opaca on the Heart. Journal of Experimental Biology and Medicine, 1931 / 06 Vol. 28; Iss. 9.

A cannula was tied in the inferior vena cava and the heart arranged for perfusion by the Symes' method, with Ringer's solution in one bottle and Ringer's solution plus the drug in the other.

The movements of the lever were recorded on a smoked drum.

The extract was prepared by macerating the dried fruit in number 20 powder with 70% alcohol for 4 days and filtering.

When required for use the alcohol was evaporated off and the thick syrupy remains added to frog Ringer's solution. Perfusion in a proportion of one part of the crude drug in 750 parts of Ringer's solution resulted in an increase in the amplitude of the beat.

Although the diastole of the heart was increased to some extent the main effect was a more complete shortening of the muscle.

After allowing the heart to return to normal by perfusing with Ringer's solution only, the above effects of the drug could be demonstrated as often as desired.

This increase in amplitude was accompanied by either a slight decrease or no change in the rate.

When the concentration of the drug was increased to one in 300 there was a marked decrease in the relaxation of the ventricle and in a short time the heart was arrested in systole; there was also a decrease in the number of impulses sent out by the sinus so that the heart was slowed.

TEN-IN= TANNIN

(sound alike)

Pancoast' found the fruit of Ilex opaca to contain tannin, pectin, albumin and 2 crystalline principles and organic salts of potassium calcium and magnesium.

Venable extracted from the leaves of the Yopon (Ilen: cmsene, Linn.) a white crystalline substance which he believed to be caffeine.

In some respects the tracings made in this work resemble those obtained by Heathcote and by Roth on perfusion of the frog's heart with the zanthine compounds.

However, on close examination there are certain features such as the systolic standstill which suggest a digitalis-like action.

An attempt to isolate the principle responsible for the characteristic effects and a more extensive investigation of the pharmacological action of the drug was being carried out.

Waud RA (1932). A digitalis-like action of extracts made from holly. J Pharmacol Exp Ther 45:27.

CONICAL ARROW HEAD WERE POISONED AMPLE

Conical arrowheads were soaked & laced with cardiotoxic poisons like aconite, conium, digitalis, oleander, Calotropis & Holly berries derived toxin, to hunt the deers in conical snow mountains, for procuring musk, the scent.

MY TOXIN ACTS LIKE DIGITALIS IN ECG TO SKEW

Experimental studies performed on frog and rabbit hearts, showed that extracts of fruits and seeds are similar in toxicity to digitalis (Waud, 1931-1932).

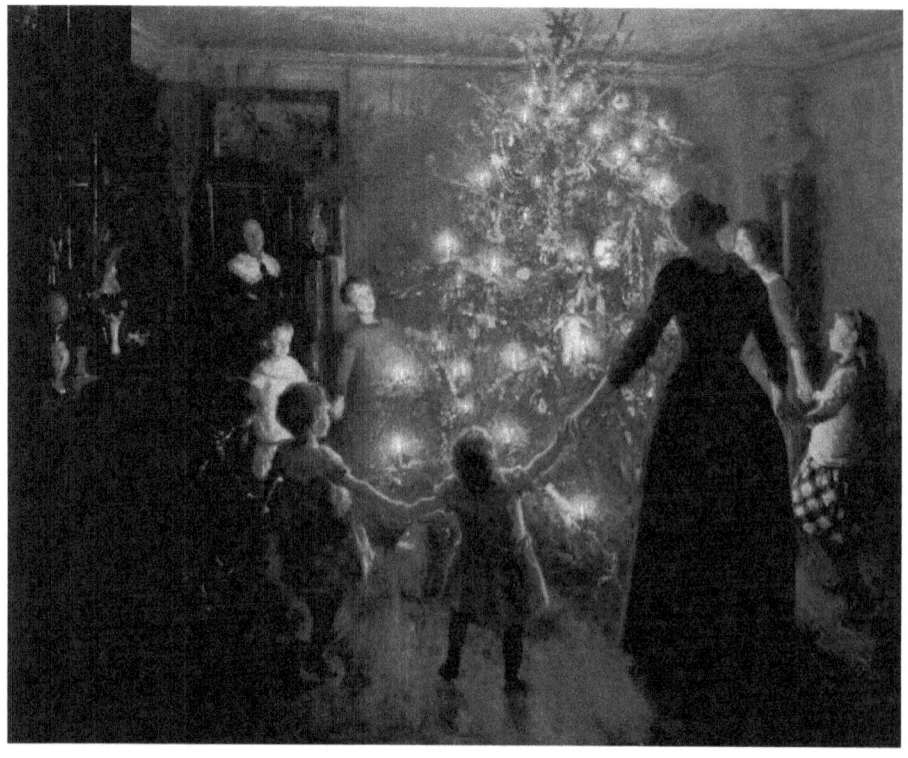

Figure 21. Christmas tree glowed by lighting Candles on branches & family dancing around to sing carols for praising Lord Jesus's birth. Image source: Viggo Johansen(1891) - The Skagen Painters: "Silent Night"

BETTER BUY MY ARTIFICIAL TREES GLOW CANDLE

Since Ilex is toxic, so its look alike artificial tree is decorated with reddish berries like balls, to represent Holly tree.

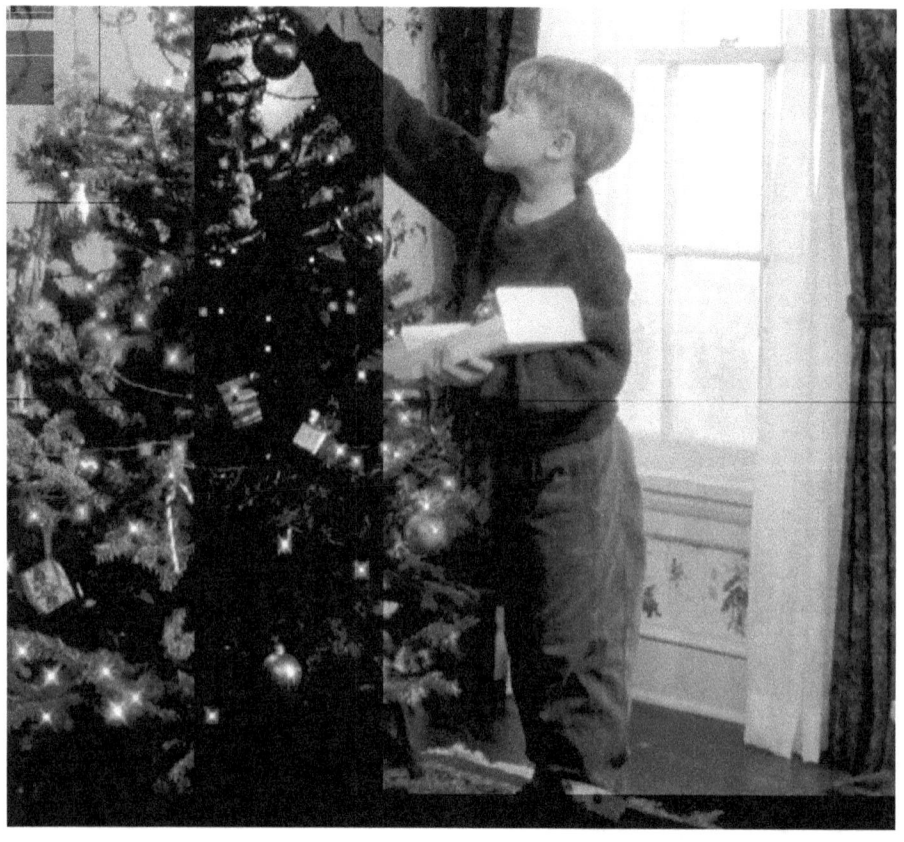

Figure 22. Movie scene from Home alone (1990) about Christmas tree decoration

AND ENJOY SAFE FESTIVALS, HAPPY YEAR, NEW

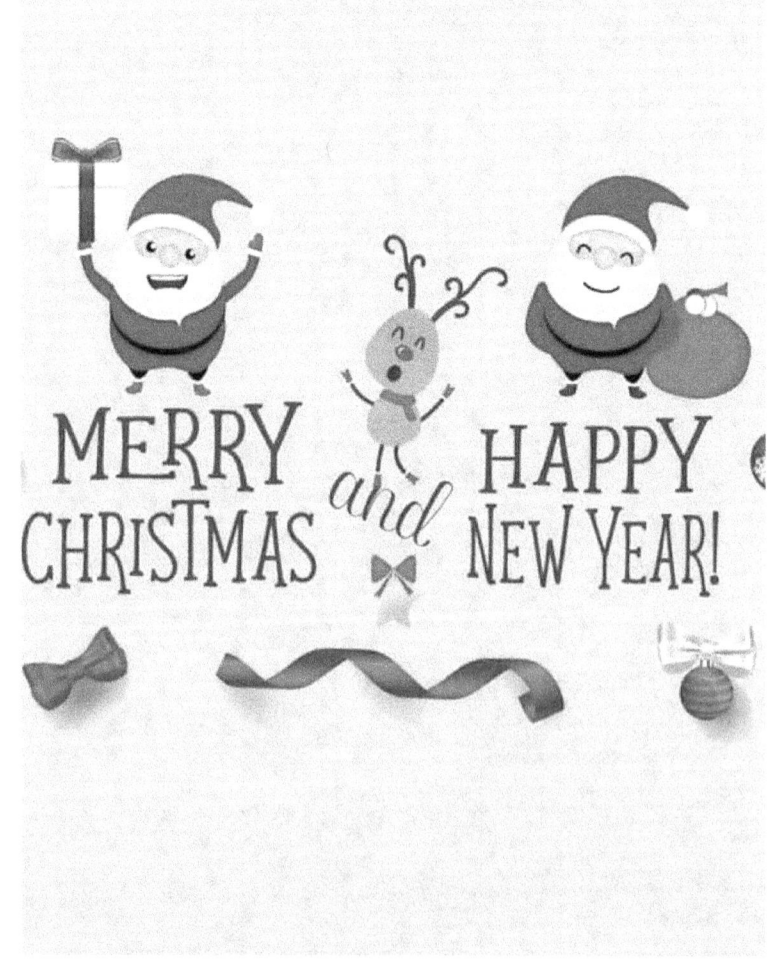

The leaves and fruit are the parts of the plant that have been used in medicine; in domestic practice alterative properties have been assigned to it and by eclectic practitioners it has been used as an anti-intermittent, febrifuge, tonic and diaphoretic.

The "Black Drink" by which the Indians "cleansed" themselves by drinking sufficient to cause vomiting was an aqueous extract prepared from the leaves of the holly.

The dried leaves of certain species of ilex are used by the inhabitants of Paraguay to prepare a stimulating beverage.

Holly is a popular winter Christmas and holiday season decoration.

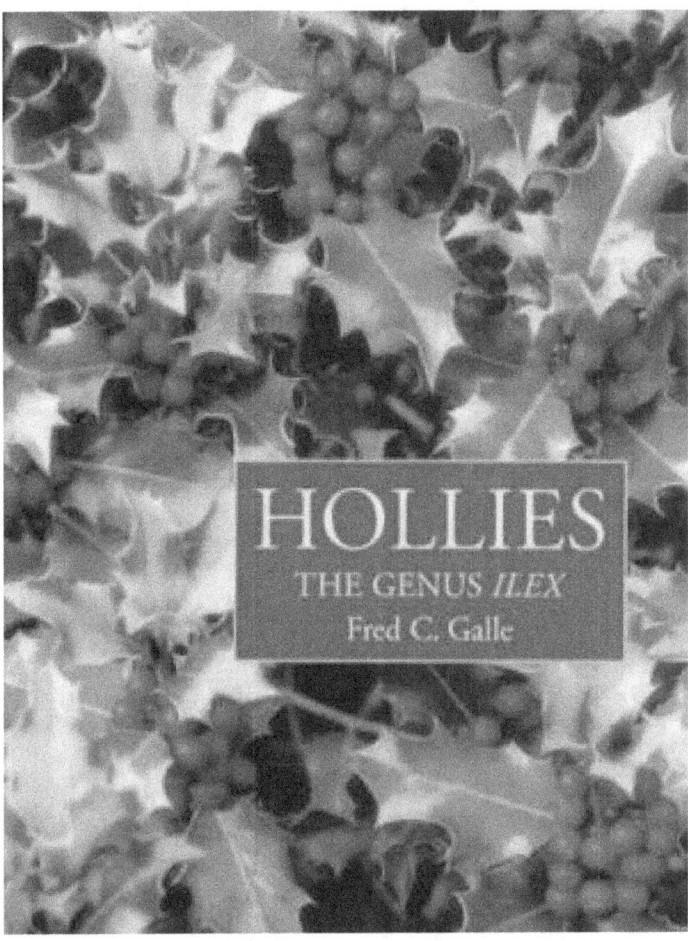

In English poetry and English stories the holly is inseparably connected with the merry-making and greetings which gather around the Christmas time.

Many poems and songs have featured the holly.

A Christmas poem in an almanac of 1695 begins:

> 'With holly and ivy so green and so gay,
> We deck up our houses as fresh as the day.'

And even King Henry VIII used holly to help describe his love for one of his many ladies in "Green Groweth the Holly" from Poetry of the English Renaissance 1509-1660.

The poem begins:

> Green groweth the holly, so doth the ivy.
> Though winter blasts blow never so high,
> Green groweth the holly.
>
> As the holly groweth green
> And never changeth hue,
> So am I, and ever hath been,
> Unto my lady true.

After reading this poem, Ilex opaca, American holly, will forever have a much more romantic meaning.

The English term Christmas ("mass on Christ's day") is of fairly recent origin.

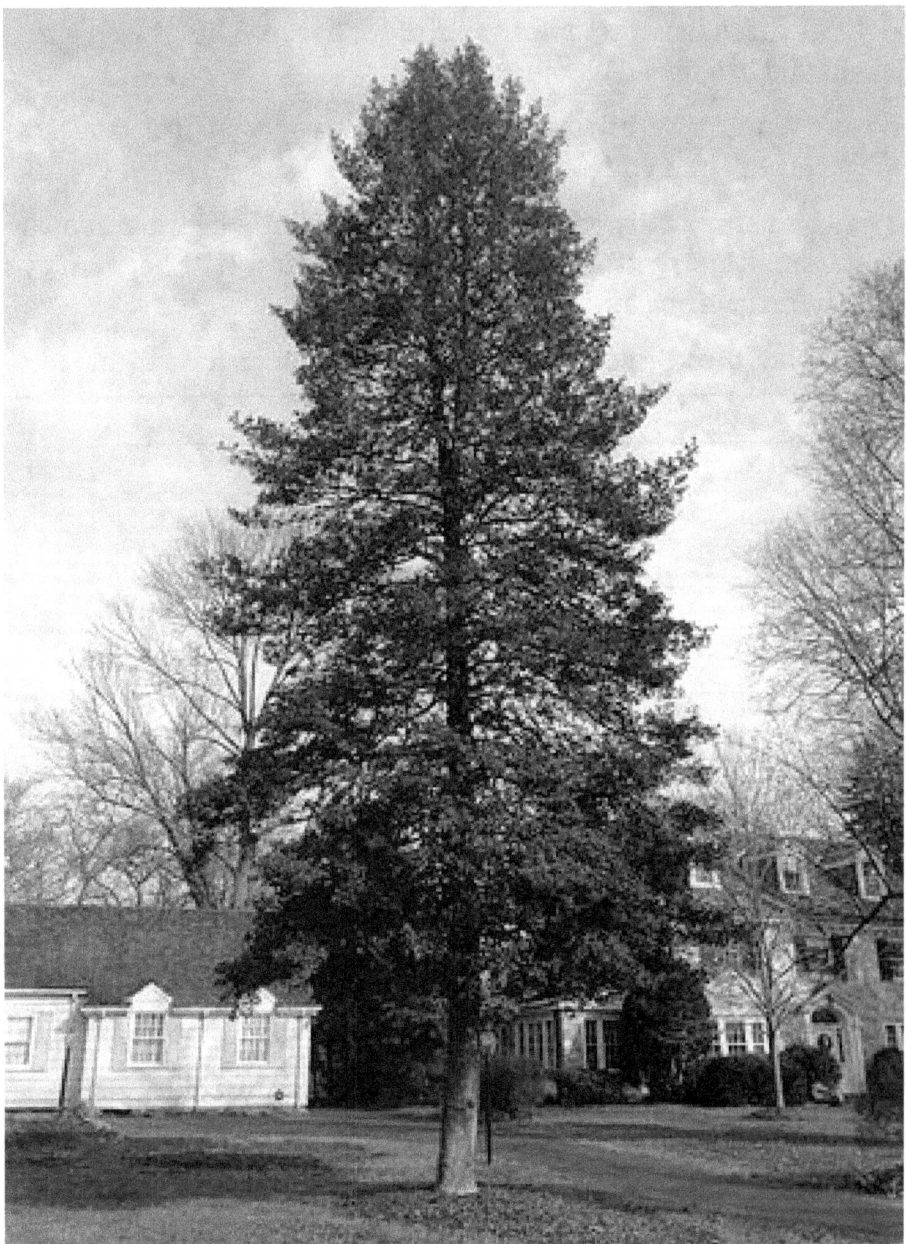

Figure 23. Pyramidal shape of Christmas Tree, Ilex Opaca

This is one of those plants that symbolizes Christmas, winter, and the holidays for many people.

Holly is often used in tabletop displays because of its rich green leaves and bright red berries.

While it can grow quite big, most people keep it trimmed back to a few feet tall and wide.

It can be a bit prickly (the leaves), which usually keeps kids away from taste-testing the berries, but you should still keep an eye out if you have one around.

By the way, birds love the berries in winter when food is scarce!

Common Name	Holly, American holly
Botanical Name	*Ilex opaca spp.*
Zone	5 to 9
Height	up to 30 feet
Spread	up to 20 feet
Foliage	Waxy green leaves and bright red berries
Light Needs	Full sun to part shade
Level of Toxicity	2
Toxic Parts	Berries

All holly berries are poisonous.

If a child or animal eats holly berries, you might witness vomiting, diarrhea, dehydration, and drowsiness.

This can occur after just a few berries, so you definitely want to take precaution if you know there have been a few (or many) eaten.

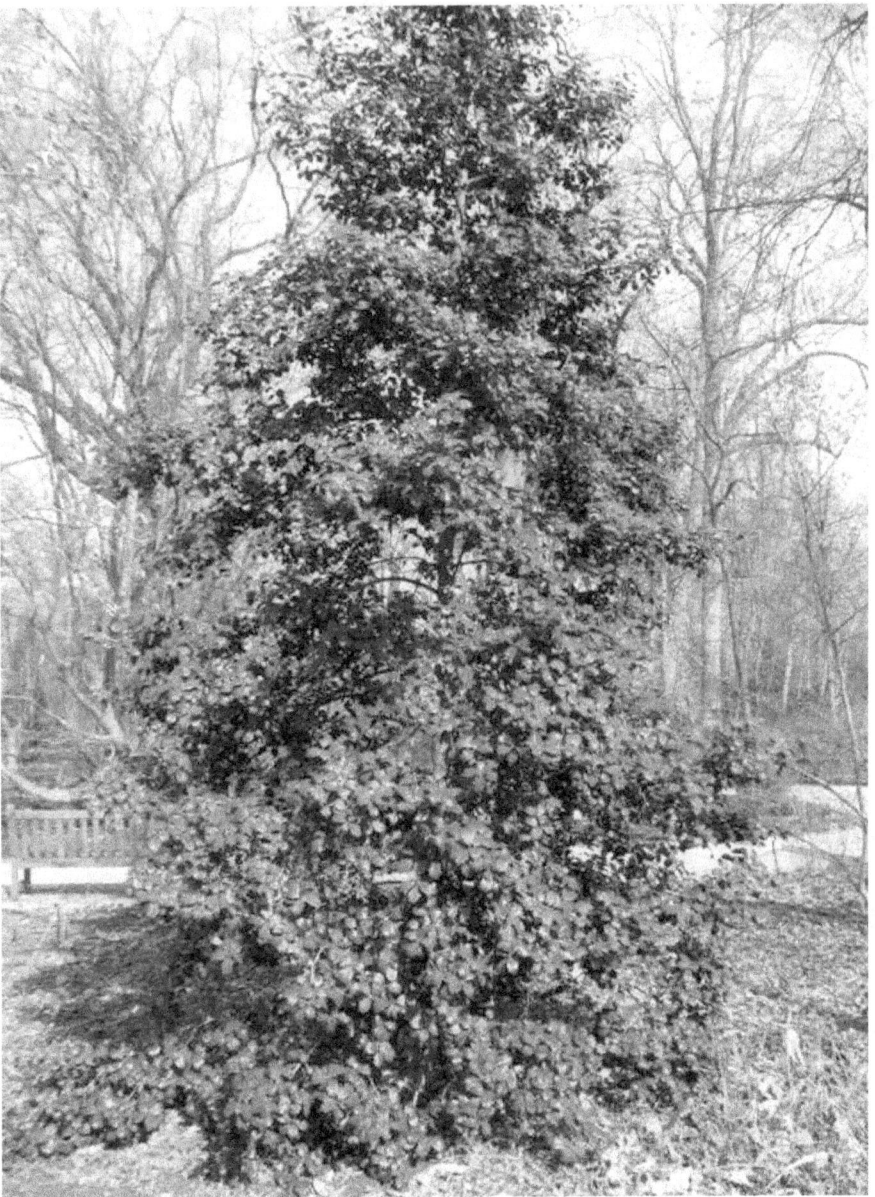

Figure 24. 'Waysides Christmas Tree' is a pyramidal tree that is noted for its dense foliage and abundant crop of deep red berries. Image source: http://www.missouribotanicalgarden.org/PlantFinder/FullImageDisplay.aspx?documentid=30035

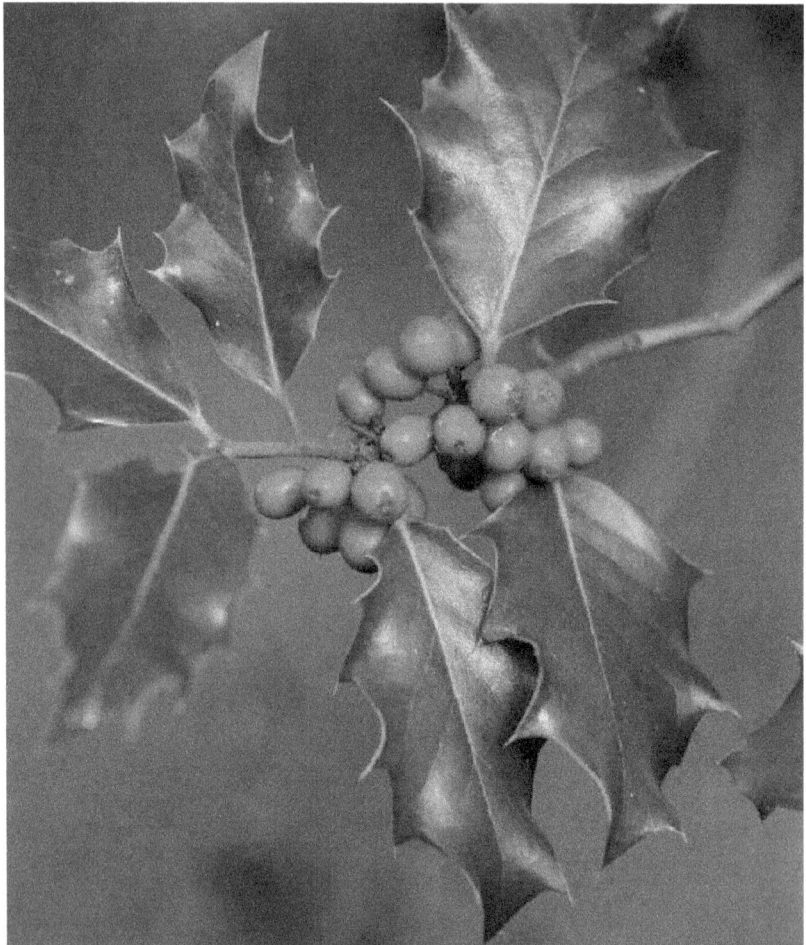

Figure 25. Ilex opaqa

This plant is called dioecious, which means male and female flowers are on different plants.

This means you'll need both a male and female if you want to get the colorful berries.

Tornio, Stacy. Plants That Can Kill 101 Toxic Species to Make You Think Twice. 2017

HOW CAN YOU TELL AN AMERICAN HOLLY FROM ENGLISH HOLLY?

Look at the color of the leaves.

English holly has a deep green color and glossy finish.

American holly leaves are a lighter, yellow-green with a dull sheen.

Variegated leaves, ever popular during the holidays, indicate English holly.

The American holly naturally grows in the deep woods, is a midstory tree, and is the state tree of Delaware.

These holly trees were noticed by the Pilgrims who landed in country the week before Christmas in 1620 on the coast of Massachusetts.

When they saw it, the American holly reminded them of their native English holly, Ilex aquifolium, which was a symbol of Christmas in England and much of Europe.

THE CHRISTMAS HOLLY POEM BY ELIZA COOK (1818-1889)

The holly! the holly! oh, twine it with bay—
Come give the holly a song;
For it helps to drive stern winter away,
With his garment so sombre and long;

It peeps through the trees with its berries of red,
And its leaves of burnished green,
When the flowers and fruits have long been dead,
And not even the daisy is seen.
Then sing to the holly, the Christmas holly,
That hangs over peasant and king;

While we laugh and carouse 'neath its glittering boughs,
To the Christmas holly we'll sing.

The gale may whistle, the frost may come
To fetter the gurgling rill;

The woods may be bare, and warblers dumb,
    But holly is beautiful still.
In the revel and light of princely halls
    The bright holly branch is found;
And its shadow falls on the lowliest walls,
    While the brimming horn goes round.

The ivy lives long, but its home must be
    Where graves and ruins are spread;
There's beauty about the cypress tree,
    But it flourishes near the dead;
The laurel the warrior's brow may wreathe,
    But it tells of tears and blood;
I sing the holly, and who can breathe
    Aught of that that is not good?
Then sing to the holly, the Christmas holly,
    That hangs over peasant and king;
While we laugh and carouse 'neath its glittering boughs,
    To the Christmas holly we'll sing.

https://en.wikisource.org/wiki/Our_American_Holidays_-_Christmas/The_Christmas_Holly

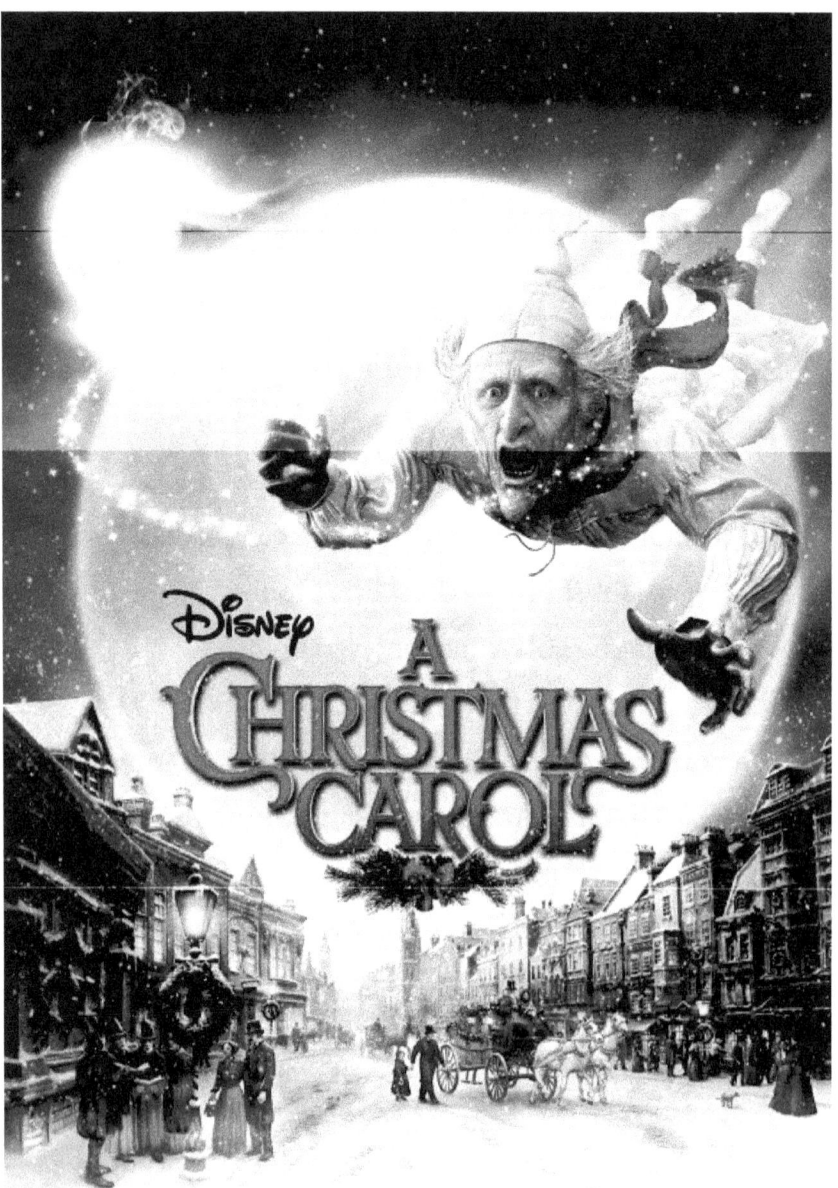

Figure 26. Hollywood movie (2009) by Walt Disney on Christmas Carol, based

on Charles Dickens novel.

CHARLES DICKENS - A CHRISTMAS CAROL

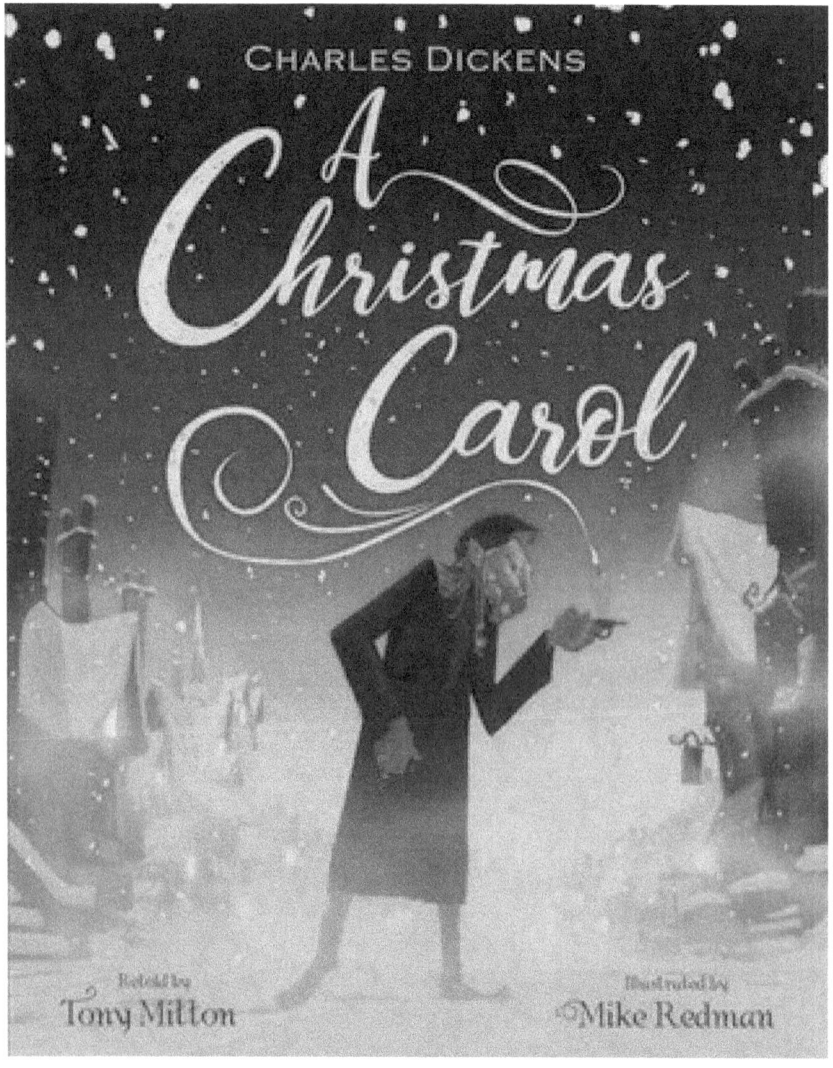

Figure 27. Charles Dickens - A Christmas Carol

Charles Dickens in 1843 novella A Christmas Carol remains especially popular and continues to inspire adaptations in every artistic genre.

In Prose. Being a Ghost Story of Christmas,

A Christmas Carol recounts the story of Ebenezer Scrooge, an elderly miser who is visited by the ghost of his former business partner Jacob Marley and the Spirits of Christmas Past, Present and Yet to Come. After their visits, Scrooge is transformed into a kinder, gentler man.

Dickens wrote A Christmas Carol during a period when the British were exploring and re-evaluating past Christmas traditions, including carols, and newer customs such as Christmas trees.

Thus Christmas Carol & Christmas Trees tradition, both became quite popular.

BIBLIOGRAPHY & SUGGESTED READING:

1) Goldfrank's Toxicological Emergencies. 11th Edition. McGraw Hills. 2015.

2) Holstege, CP. Toxicology Recall. 1st Ed. LWW. 2010.

3) Modi. Medical Jurisprudence & Toxicology. 26th Edition. Lexis Nexis. 2018

4) Kulkarni, ML. Pediatric Toxicology. 1st Ed. Paras Publishers. 2010.

5) Pillay, VV. Practical Medicolegal Manual. 1st Ed. Paras Publishers. 2019.

6) Tiwari, Satish. Textbook of Medicolegal issues. 2nd Edition. 2018.

7) Biswas, G. Recent Advances in Forensic Medicine & Toxicology. Vol.2. Jaypee. 2018.

8) Richhariya, D. Textbook of Emergency & trauma care. 1st ed. Jaypee. 2018.

9) Kanchan, Tanuj. Rapid Review of Toxicology. 1st ed. Jaypee. 2018.

10) Agarwal, Praveen. Diagnosis & management of Common poisoning. Oxford 1st ed. OUP. 1998.

11) Olson, K. Poisoning & Drug Overdose. 7th Ed. McGrawHills. 2018.

12) Knight, Bernard. Forensic Pathology. 4th Edition. CRC Press. 2018.

13) WHO (World Health Organisation) Guidelines for the management of snake-bites in South-East Asia. 2016.

14) Singh, Omendra. Priniciple & Practice of Critical Care Toxicology. 1st ed. Jaypee. 2019.

15) Grover, JK. Diagnosis & Management of Poisoning. 1st Ed. Peepee. 2006.

16) Pillay, VV. Modern Medical Toxicology. 4th ed. Jaypee. 2016.

17) Grover, A. Pocketbook of Poisoning. 1st ed. Pushpanjili publishers. 2006.

18) Devarajan, TV. Diagnosis & Treatment of Poisoning & Drug overdose Made Easy. 1st Ed. Jaypee. 2015.

19) Pillay, VV. Comprehensive Medical Toxicology. 3rd ed. Paras Medical Publishers. 2018.

OUR BOOKS ON TOXICOLOGY

1. Verma, Vivekanshu. Shankar, S., Bansal, A. Critical Care Nursing in Emergency Toxicology. 1st Ed. Redflower publishers.2019. https://www.amazon.in/Critical-Care-Nursing-Emergency-Toxicology/dp/8194255023/

2. Verma, Vivekanshu. Toxi-Comic Series: Toxic Emergencies. 1st Ed. Scholar's Press. Germany. Online Link : https://www.amazon.com/dp/6138837347/ref=rdr_ext_tmb

3. Verma, Vivekanshu. Venugopalan, P. Kochar SR. Toxicological Emergencies - A to Z Encyclopedia of Poison & Antidotes. 1st Ed. Scholar's Press. Germany.

Online Link: https://www.amazon.fr/Toxicological-EmergenciesEncyclopaedia-Toxicologist-ToxicoLegal/dp/3639760298

4. Verma, Vivekanshu. Kochar SR, Richhariya, D. Managing Toxicological Emergencies Made Ridiculously Funny for Doctors. 1st Ed. Scholar's Press. Germany. 2019. Online Link : https://www.amazon.com/Managing-Toxicological-Emergencies-Ridiculously-Doctors/dp/6138830954

5. Verma, Vivekanshu. Kochar SR, Richhariya, D. Practical Workbook Emergency Trauma & Toxicology in Simulation Training. 1st Edition,2019 . Published by Redflower Publications, New Delhi

https://www.amazon.in/Practical-Emergency-Toxicology-Workbook-Simulation/dp/8193073568/

6. Verma, Vivekanshu. Pillay VV. Kochar SR. Medical Toxicology Life Support Skills Learning by Simulation Training. 1st Ed. Scholar's Press, Germany.2019.

Online Link: https://www.amazon.com/Medical-Toxicology-Learning-Simulation-

Training/dp/6202317868/

7. Venkatram, Bhat, S. Matre, Madulika. Verma, Vivekanshu. Sirur. Textbook of Medicolegal issues in Plastic surgery & Dermatology, 1st Edition. Jaypee publishers. Delhi. Online Link:http://www.jaypeebrothers.com/pgDetails.aspx?cat=s&book_id=9789352708970

8. Verma, Vivekanshu. Jena, N. Senthilkumaran, Pillay, VV. ISTOLS Course Material for High-Fidelity Simulation Training in Managing Poisoning, Intoxication & Drug Overdose. 1st ed. Published by Indian Society of Toxicology, AIMS, Kochi.2017

9. Verma, Vivekanshu. Shankar, S., Bansal, A. Toxicology Nurse.1st Ed. Scholar's Press.2019

Link:https://www.morebooks.de/store/gb/book/toxicology-nurse-:-critical-care-nursing-in-toxicological-emergencies/isbn/978-613-8-91091-6

10. Saxena, V. Manickam, S. Verma, Vivekanshu. Legal & Forensic Importance of Human Anatomy: Evidence based Cases. 1st Ed. Scholar's Press. Link: https://www.bookdepository.com/Legal-Forensic-Importance-Human-Anatomy-Evidence-based-Cases-Vivekanshu-Verma/9786138915171

11. Verma, Vivekanshu.. Kochar SR. Rastogi, P. OSCE & OSPE in Clinical Toxicology 1st Ed. Scholar's Press. Germany. Online Link: https://www.morebooks.shop/book-price_offer_fe61704277678f1c0c004b7129b7bcaf899a9164?locale=gb&currency=EUR

12. Verma, V. Pillay, VV. Kochar SR. Rastogi, P. Toxic Riddles by Toxic Detective- Volume One. Kindle Edition. 2020. Amazon Link: https://www.amazon.in/dp/B08D952NDZ

13. Verma, V. Pillay, VV. Kochar SR. Rastogi, P. Toxic Riddles by Toxic Detective- Volume Two. Kindle Edition. 2020. Amazon Link: https://www.amazon.in/dp/B08GBYT9TR

14. Verma, V. Pillay, VV. Kochar SR. Rastogi, P. Toxic Riddles by Toxic Detective- Volume Three. Kindle Edition. 2020. Amazon Link: https://www.amazon.in/dp/

B08GG7L7Q3

15. Verma, V. Pillay, VV. Kochar SR. Rastogi, P. Current Protocols in Medical Toxicology: Indian Society of Toxicology Initiative. Kindle Edition. 2020. Amazon Link: https://www.amazon.in/dp/B08HK2RQ5N

16. Verma, V. Pillay, VV. Kochar SR. Rastogi, P. Calotropis : Toxic Riddles by Toxic Detective. Kindle Edition. 2020. Amazon Link: https://www.amazon.in/dp/B08HJTGZ7P

17. Verma, V. Pillay, VV. Kochar SR. Rastogi, P. Neem: Toxic Riddles by Toxic Detective. Kindle Edition. 2020. Amazon Link: https://www.amazon.in/dp/B08HVWJ6QG

18. Verma, V. Pillay, VV. Kochar SR. Rastogi, P. ACE Inhibitors: Toxic Riddles by Toxic Detective. Kindle Edition. 2020. Amazon Kindle Link: https://www.amazon.in/dp/B08JB2251K

19. Verma, V. Pillay, VV. Kochar SR. Rastogi, P. Death camas: Toxic Riddles by Toxic Detective. Kindle Edition. 2020. Amazon Link: https://www.amazon.in/dp/B08JS9PHKB

20. Verma, V. Pillay, VV. Kochar SR. Rastogi, P. Novichok: Toxic Riddles by Toxic Detective. Kindle Edition. 2020. Amazon Link: https://www.amazon.com/dp/B08K3WF2D4

21. Verma, V. Pillay, VV. Kochar SR. Rastogi, P. MAHUA: Toxic Riddles by Toxic Detective. Kindle Edition. 2020. Amazon Link: https://www.amazon.in/dp/B08KCG1YXY

22. Verma, V. Pillay, VV. Kochar SR. Rastogi, P. Poison Damsels: Toxic Riddles by Toxic Detective. Kindle Edition. 2020. Amazon Link: https://www.amazon.in/dp/B08L41TW1D

23. Verma, V. Pillay, VV. Kochar SR. Rastogi, P. Patel, SH. Corrosive Burns: Toxic Riddles by Toxic Detective. Kindle Edition. 2020. Amazon Link: https://www.amazon.com/dp/B08L3XBWRT

24. Verma, V. Pillay, VV. Kochar SR. Rastogi, P. Patel, SH. *Analyzing Toxicology: Toxic Riddles by Toxic Detective.* Kindle Edition. 2020. Amazon Link: https://www.amazon.in/dp/B08MBDBPGW

25. Verma, V. Pillay, VV. Kochar SR. Rastogi, P. Patel, SH. *Arum family of Araceae: Toxic Riddles by Toxic Detective.* Kindle Edition. 2020. Amazon Link: https://www.amazon.in/dp/B08N496RWD

26. Verma, V. Pillay, VV. Kochar SR. Rastogi, P. Patel, SH. *Methyl Isocyanate MIC: Toxic Riddles by Toxic Detective.* Kindle Edition. 2020. Amazon Link: https://www.amazon.in/dp/B08M5N7HZM

27. Verma, V. Pillay, VV. Kochar SR. Rastogi, P. Patel, SH. *Dwarf Lark Spur: Toxic Riddles by Toxic Detective.* Kindle Edition. 2020. Amazon Link: https://www.amazon.in/dp/B08N8L2J57

28. Verma, V. Pillay, VV. Kochar SR. Rastogi, P. Patel, SH. *Passion flower & Fruit: Toxic Riddles by Toxic Detective.* Kindle Edition. 2020. Amazon Link : https://www.amazon.in/dp/B08NKBMJ8J

29. Verma, V. Pillay, VV. Kochar SR. Rastogi, P. Patel, SH. *One, Four- Butanediol: Toxic Riddles by Toxic Detective.* Kindle Edition. 2020. Amazon Link: https://www.amazon.in/dp/B08P59RKGY

30. Verma, V. Pillay, VV. Kochar SR. Rastogi, P. Panwar, V. *Sweet Flag Calamus: Toxic Riddles by Toxic Detective.* Kindle Edition. 2020. Amazon Link: https://www.amazon.com/dp/B08PG183S5

31. Verma, V. Pillay, VV. Kochar SR. Rastogi, P. Panwar, V. *Asphaltum Punjabinum: Toxic Riddles by Toxic Detective.* Kindle Edition. 2020. Amazon Link: https://www.amazon.com/dp/B08PTXW378

31. Verma, V. Pillay, VV. Kochar SR. Rastogi, P. Panwar, V. *Mystery of the Musk: Toxic Riddles by Toxic Detective.* Kindle Edition. 2020. Amazon Link: https://www.amazon.com/dp/B08QW5RM1K

CONTRIBUTORS:

1. Dr Yatin Mehta, Chairman, Anaesthesia, Critical Care, Emergency & Trauma care, Medanta-The Medicity, Gurugram

2. Dr P Venugopalan, Director, Emergency & Trauma care, MIMS, Calicut

3. Mr Santosh Kumar Verma, Senior Advocate, Rajasthan High Court

4. Dr Tariq Ali, Director, Critical Care, Medanta-The Medicity, Gurugram

5. Dr Praveen Aggarwal, Professor & Head, Department of Emergency Medicine, AIIMS, New Delhi

6. Dr Venkat Raghav, Professor & HOD, Forensic Medicine & toxicology, Bangalore Medical College, Bengaluru.

7. Dr Ajay Gangele, Professor, Forensic Medicine & Toxicology, DY Patil Medical college, Pune

8. Dr Krishnadutt Chavali, Professor, Forensic Medicine & Toxicology, AIIMS, Raipur

9. Dr SK Singhal, Professor &HOD, Forensic Medicine & Toxicology, Ananta Institute of Medical sciences and research center, Rajsamand (Rajasthan).

10. Dr Dhruv Chaudhary, Senior Professor & Head, Pulmonary & Critical Care Medicine, PGIMS, Rohtak

11. Dr Tejas Prajapati, Consultant Toxicologist, AMC MET Medical College, Ahmedabad, Gujarat

12. Dr Karen Harshita, Senior Resident, Forensic Medicine & Toxicology, Bangalore medical College and research institute, Bangalore

13. Dr Ajith Antony Senior Resident, Forensic Medicine & Toxicology, Goa

14. Dr Lishu Chaure, Senior Resident, Palamu Medical College, Palamu Jharkhand.

15. Dr Somashekar Chandren, Assistant professor Forensic Medicine & Toxicology, AIMS, B G Nagara, Mandya, Karnataka

16. Dr Latif Johnson, Assistant professor, Forensic Medicine & Toxicology, Chris-

tain Medical College, Vellore

17. Dr Arjit Dey, Senior Resident, Forensic Medicine & Toxicology, AIIMS, Delhi

18. Dr Kashif Ali, Senior Resident, Forensic Medicine & Toxicology, Jawaharlal Nehru Medical College, AMU, Aligarh (UP)

19. Dr. Shweta H Patel, Assistant Professor, Forensic Medicine & Toxicology, Pramukhswami Medical College, Karamsad. Dist. Anand, Gujarat.

20. Dr Suman K. Charawati, Scientist, Forensic Science Lab, Assam

21. Dr Walter Waz, Professor, Forensic Medicine & Toxicology, Mumbai

22. Dr Vatsal Pawnar, BAMS, Diploma in Cosmetology, Ayurvedic Cosmetologist, Gurugram

23. Dr Vidusha Vijay, Forensic Medicine & Toxicology Consultant, Columbia Asia Hospital Bangalore

24. R. R. Rajitha, Emergency Nursing officer, King Faisal Hospital, Riyadh, Saudi Arabia

www.ingramcontent.com/pod-product-compliance
Lightning Source LLC
Chambersburg PA
CBHW060843220526
45466CB00003B/1217